Outliving Your Ovaries

An Endocrinologist Weighs the Risks and Rewards of
Treating Menopause with Hormone Replacement Therapy

Marina Johnson, M.D., F.A.C.E.

EYESONG
PUBLISHING

OUTLIVING YOUR OVARIES
An Endocrinologist Weighs The Risks And Rewards
Of Treating Menopause With Hormone Replacement Therapy

PUBLISHED BY
EYESONG PUBLISHING
Irving, Texas
www.EyesongPublishing.com

Library of Congress Control Number: 2011904697
ISBN ISBN 10 1461018781
ISBN 13 978-1461018780

This book is available at quantity discounts for bulk purchases.
For more information, call Gordon Blocker, 214-770-2330.

Praise for the Book

Outliving Your Ovaries

"Finally-a clear concise prescription for women as they navigate the challenges of menopause. Debunking misconceptions, Dr. Johnson provides a roadmap for health and vitality in what can be truly golden years."

Catherine Crier
Journalist, former Judge and best-selling Author

"Women who read Outliving Your Ovaries and use the information to take estrogen will enhance the quality and quantity of their lives."

Daniel R. Mishell, Jr., M.D.
Professor Emeritus, Obstetrics & Gynecology
University of Southern California
School of Medicine
Associate Editor
Journal of Reproductive Medicine

"I believe this book will be a great benefit to women who are struggling in the area of hormonal imbalance. Dr. Johnson explains the difference between synthetic hormones and natural hormone replacement therapy. So many women are struggling with their hormones, hot flashes, mood swings, etc. Dr. Johnson brings her years of experience to answer women's questions and gives practical solutions that address the root of the problem versus treating the symptom! A must read for all women. Dr. Johnson takes great care to deal with each of her patients on an individual basis. I appreciate her thoroughness in testing, studying your medical history and taking time to put the pieces of your health puzzle together. She has provided excellent care for me and my family."

Joni Lamb
Co-Founder, Daystar Television Network

"This is a must read for any woman perimenopausal or menopausal. You will be filled with the knowledge to make educated choices about how you want to feel. The book is written as if you were in the office with Dr. Marina Johnson herself. She has a way of making complicated medical terms and conditions easy to understand. She takes away the fear created by media sound bite about woman's hormones and educates you with the real facts. I can't wait to give this book to my women friends and have them be able to benefit from it as much as I have from being a patient of Dr. Johnson's for several years. I feel great...thanks to Dr. Johnson and you can too!"

Cindy Waldrip
Patient

"Dr. Marina Johnson has been my primary physician for well over ten years. As a business woman, a sharp mind is critical to being successful. And as a grandmother, being able to crawl through the tunnels of Chuck E. Cheese with my grand kids and play a mean game of softball with them, is priceless. I can honestly thank Dr. Johnson for that. Her approach to wellness and preventive care has kept me in top shape both mentally and physically. I have been privileged to review 'Outliving Your Ovaries'. It is filled with such important information that when I finished reading it, I asked Dr. Johnson to save five copies. I want my daughters and daughters-in-laws to each have a copy. All are in their thirties and forties and need to read this extraordinary book."

Barbara
Patient

" 'Outliving Your Ovaries' is a well written book that will help empower women to make educated choices about the use of postmenopausal hormone therapy."

Alan M. Altman, M.D.
Medical Coordinator "Hot Flash Havoc" - the Movie
President
International Society for the Study of Women's Sexual Health
(ISSWSH)

"'Outliving Your Ovaries' is a book that should interest every member of the human race, including men. Most men have women in their lives (I have a wife, daughter, mother, sister, cousins, etc.) and most women have men in their lives who care about them. Women have a unique biology that I never understood before reading Dr. Johnson's book. Women need to understand that even making 'no decision' about replacing female hormones carries consequences! Dr. Johnson's book bridges the huge knowledge gaps between the lay person and the pharmaceutical industry, between hype and the facts, between the lay person and medical researchers, between sound bite news reports and detailed medical analysis of studies and between patients and treating physicians. Her passion for patient care comes through on every page of the book and every word focuses on giving her menopausal patients and the physicians who treat them, the medical knowledge necessary to allow them to live long, productive, vigorous and healthy lives. Any woman approaching perimenopause or menopause and any man who cares for such a woman, should arm themselves with the knowledge provided by Dr. Johnson's book."

Mark W. Walker
Attorney

"This is an incredible book to learn about your body, its hormonal changes and to arm yourself with much needed information to be smart about your health and healthcare"

Natasha Naquin
Advertising Executive

" 'Outliving Your Ovaries' is an excellent, comprehensive resource on hormone therapy for women considering this as an option. Medical decision making should be made as a collaboration between the physician and a well informed patient. This book will help address many of the key questions that form the basis for deciding on what therapy options are most appropriate based on clinical judgment for each woman as an individual."

Steven M. Petak M.D., J.D., F.A.C.E.
Associate
Texas Institute for Reproductive Medicine and Endocrinology
Houston, Texas

"This book should end much of the confusion around menopause. It will get the conversation out in the open. It will wake up many women about the consequences of aging. We all strive to regain the vigor and mental alertness we had before menopause. Dr. Johnson provides the basis for a meaningful conversation with your doctor about treating menopausal symptoms as a disorder that can be corrected. It sheds light on the risks of not treating hormone deficiencies in addition to interpreting the studies that show some risks of taking certain types of hormone replacements. It's written by a widely experienced endocrinologist with a commitment to helping women live the fullest healthiest lives possible as they age. The language is easily understood in layman terms and does not bog down in excessive medical jargon.

For me as a patient - She has recommended treatments that have completely solved a list of issues that cropped up during and after menopause. I first went to see her about pelvic pain during intercourse. Not expecting more than to solve that one issue I have been pleasantly surprised by many other benefits. In less than 5 months her customized prescriptions for HRT not only solved vaginal atrophy issues common in menopausal women but I have also been successful in weaning off of medications for mild high blood pressure (Lisinopril) and athletic asthma (Advair inhaler). In addition, I no longer need the daily 1 hour afternoon naps to supplement my nightly 8-9 hours sleep just to get through the day and my memory is sharper than before I started treatments. I am no longer taking the high risk drug, Prempro, for HRT as she has replaced it with safer and much more effective bioidentical hormones using transdermal delivery.

No one wants to talk about how bad sex can get as you age. Aging men get the advantage of buying ED drugs for enhanced recreation but what about their aging partner? I found that the pain during intercourse completely killed my libido. Once the pain was solved my interest in sex returned to normal. My husband is much happier too."

L.G.E.
Patient

"I had a hysterectomy when I was 46 years old and was prescribed Premarin as a hormone replacement by my doctor. Because my mother died of breast cancer and I had read many articles relating to hormones and breast cancer, I opted not to take the Premarin. I lived the night sweats,

adult acne and decreased libido/vaginal dryness - but thought that was better to endure than the chance of breast cancer. (My husband was not so convinced.) Heck, I was emotionally balanced, slept great, and had plenty of energy - so what could possibly be wrong.

It wasn't until my normally perfect (even on the low side) blood pressure was off the charts did I decide to take my friend's advice and see Dr. Marina Johnson. I was so impressed at the time she took to know me and my physical-emotional-spiritual history. I will admit, I was a little surprised at the thoroughness of her testing.

Dr. Johnson convinced me that my blood pressure problems were far more dangerous than the threat of breast cancer. She began a gradual building of a balanced hormone replacement for me. During my visits to her office, I had the chance to read 'Outliving Your Ovaries' as it was a lengthy work in progress. In every chapter, I saw some of my symptoms and those of friends. I highly recommend this book and a balanced hormone plan!"

Pam Minick
Television Personality

"A copy of 'Outliving Your Ovaries' is a must-have for every woman you know and care about. It is that important! Women's quality of life has suffered too long because of scarce, fragmented, incomplete bits of information that exist about our health. Dr. Johnson's life-long mission has been to seek out, study, question, observe and connect the dots correctly in an accessible manner. Her work and 'Outliving Your Ovaries' changes things! And you will immediately understand how when you read the book. And I speak from personal experience!"

Kim Young
President
the forest & the trees

"Dr. Marina Johnson is uniquely skilled in navigating the treacherous combat zone of the midlife maladies known as MENOPAUSE. Her groundbreaking research, leading-edge treatments and philosophy allow women to go through this phase of their lives with dignity and hormonal balance. As a professional woman, I survived without losing my femininity and joy of life...you can too. Thank you Dr. Marina, for touching my life."

Anne L. Holland, CEO
Mayco Petroleum, Inc.

"Dr. Marina Johnson's book 'Outliving Your Ovaries' is an absolute must read for all adult females. The Johnson Menopause Method is evidence-based and backed up by years of clinical experience. Her advice is anchored in science and delivered in a personalized manner. She tackles a very controversial subject with logic that is easy to understand. This book brings clarity to the menopausal hormone replacement therapy issue. Dr. Johnson delivers her opinions in a very objective scientifically based manner. Her thoughts are laid out in a manner that's logical and understandable for both medical providers as well as the lay public. Her willingness to share her wealth of knowledge is commendable. Her book arms women with essential information that will allow them to take responsibility for their own well being. Any adult female who reads this book will be much better prepared to deal with the hormonal changes of menopause. Dr. Johnson will enhance the lives of millions of women with her book. Healthcare providers who deliver hormone replacement therapy should be required to read this book."

Dr. Bradley F. Bale
Co-Founder of the Bale/Doneen Method
Assistant Clinical Professor
Texas Tech School of Medicine

"I've been a patient of Dr. Johnson's for 3 years now. Lousy quality of life, fat, frumpy and miserable when I found her, she has changed my life. I now love living, have lost 40 pounds, feel and look 30 years younger and only intend to get better. You owe it to yourself and the women in your life to read this book. Following her program is not easy or quick, but it's well worth the time and effort you spend. I'll never go back to the way I was. There are two most important women in my life: my mother, who gave me life; and Dr. Marina Johnson, who made it worth living again."

Celia D. Trimble

"Dr. Marina Johnson has been the personal physician for my wife, Susan and myself for the last nine years. I am 61 years old and Susan is 62. During this time, Dr. Johnson has provided us with a level of health care that can only be characterized as extraordinary. She takes the time to listen and explain and she does this in a manner that is clear and concise. She has tailored a health management program personalized for our individual needs and as a result, Susan and I are very healthy and vigorous for our age.

I graduated from college with a degree in pre-med but chose to pursue the world of business. I have owned or co-owned several companies, including one that went public on the NYSE in 1996. I am an educated health consumer and I research and learn about health issues that are affecting Susan and me. I have learned from the business world that true talent is rare. There are perhaps only 1% in any given field that are truly the best at what they do and Dr. Johnson is part of this elite group.

Dr. Johnson's approach to menopause management has enabled Susan to enjoy a better quality of life and productivity. We both travel all over the world and have great energy. I commend Dr. Johnson for sharing her knowledge and experience in her book, 'Outliving Your Ovaries', so other women can also improve their health."

Bill and Susan Casner
CEO and Entrepreneur

Contents

Dedication

This book is dedicated to my dear mother, Marina Marmolejo Gonzalez. My mother was a tiny woman at just five feet tall but she ruled our household with an iron hand. She was a very strict disciplinarian and each of the five children were expected to do their part to help out with household duties.

What my parents lacked in financial security was more than exceeded by giving us love and teaching us important attributes of self-reliance, honesty, respect for others and always doing your best - great values that helped us all acquire college degrees and achieve success in various professions.

Thank you Mom for always believing in me and for being a role model of how to live your elder years.

About the author

Marina Johnson, M.D., F.A.C.E. is the Founder and Medical Director of the Institute of Endocrinology and Preventive Medicine located in Irving, a suburb of Dallas, Texas. The mission of the Institute is to engage the patient in the active pursuit of optimal health and to provide personalized superlative care with an emphasis on preventive medicine and healthy aging. Dr. Johnson is board-certified in endocrinology and metabolism and in internal medicine. While she has a special interest in menopause, she also treats patients with disorders related to thyroid, growth hormone, premenstrual syndrome (PMS), testosterone, and prevention of diabetes and cardiovascular disease.

Dr. Johnson earned her undergraduate degree in Pharmacy from the University of Houston. She then became Assistant Editor of the *American Hospital Formulary Service-Drug Information (AHFS-DI)*, a drug reference book published by the American Society of Hospital Pharmacists. *AHFS-DI* is a non-commercial drug compendium with a long-standing record in evidence-based evaluation of information on drug use. It's been officially adopted by the US Public Health Service and recommended by the American College of Physicians as part of a library for internists. She researched the medical literature and prepared comprehensive monographs on each drug.

Dr. Johnson earned her MD from the University of California at Los Angeles and completed an internal medicine residency at UCLA/St. Mary's Medical Center in Long Beach, California. She completed her fellowship in endocrinology and metabolism at the University of Southern California in Los Angeles.

After two years at the City of Hope research hospital she returned to Texas. After one year at Kaiser Permanente in Dallas, she set up her private medical practice.

In writing **Outliving Your Ovaries**, Dr. Johnson has utilized her skills as an endocrinologist, pharmacist, and medical writer to research over 450 articles from mainstream peer-reviewed medical journals so that women and their physicians can see there is a sound, scientific basis for her recommendations. With no financial ties to any pharmaceutical company, her allegiance is to her patients and providing them unbiased information based on her clinical experience, continuing medical education and her review of the literature. Because patient education is a major focus of her practice, she's able to explain complex issues in terms most women can understand. She gives poignant patient stories from over two decades of clinical experience that enable readers to relate to the material and provides further clinical relevance to the book. Armed with this information, a woman can be in a better position to consult with her own physician and decide if hormone replacement therapy is right for her.

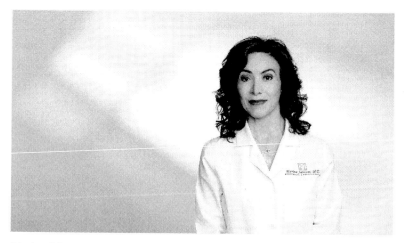

Marina Johnson, M.D., F.A.C.E

Preface

Menopause is Often Not Given Priority as a Health Problem

Because every woman goes through menopause, it's often not even considered a medical problem. In the past, women were often patted on the head and told *"Honey, you're getting older and you just need to accept it."* Today's postmenopausal women are more empowered and do not want to be placated with such condescending attitudes.

Estrogen deficiency leads to a myriad of symptoms that affect a woman's quality of life and to an increased risk of degenerative diseases including heart disease, osteoporosis, Alzheimer's disease, diabetes and colon cancer. Most of these symptoms and degenerative disorders can be either resolved or reduced with appropriate estrogen therapy. Why would we NOT want to treat and prevent such potentially serious health problems? While estrogen carries some risks, our goal should be to select therapies which give us the most benefit with the least risks. You deserve to know the facts so you can knowingly participate in this decision with you own physician.

Menopause is Treated by Primary Care Physicians Rather than Endocrinologists

While most hormones are prescribed by endocrinologists, hormone replacement therapy (HRT) is more often prescribed by obstetrician-gynecologists and family doctors. Each of these specialties focuses on a wide, extensive range of chronic problems. Since menopause is often regarded as an entity that occurs in all women and there are no menopausal "emergencies," it is often not given a high priority of importance.

Combine that view of the condition to the negative outcomes reported by the Women's Health Initiative (WHI) from the use of Prempro and Premarin, the HRT most commonly prescribed by primary care physicians and it is easy to see why 80% of postmenopausal women go untreated. In addition, there is a relative shortage of endocrinologists and most are mainly involved in treating diabetes, a growing health care issue. So there are not enough endocrinologists in practice to manage all menopausal women.

Everyone seems to be prescribing bioidentical hormone therapy these days. I have often been asked, *"How is your method for bioidentical HRT different than everyone else?"* My method is based on sound principles first introduced to me in medical school and further refined and updated by new clinical studies and the clinical responses I have seen in my patients. Since 1986, I have managed over 100,000 female patient visits, and carefully monitored estradiol blood levels in all those patients, I've been able to see which therapies are most effective and at what levels most symptoms resolve. At this point in my career, I feel the need to share this wealth of information I've learned for the purpose of improving the lives of millions of women who are depriving themselves of hormone therapy because of fear. It has been a fascinating journey and before launching into the book, I will outline my basic methodology and how I arrived at my method.

Johnson Menopause Method™

My training as an endocrinologist, my background as a former pharmacist and assistant editor for a drug reference book, and my years of clinical experience have enabled me to to develop a method that I feel is better than the current standard of care. I have stayed abreast of new medical developments by ongoing review of the literature and by attending an average of 65+ hours of annual continuing medical education. I have NO conflicts of interests or financial ties to big Pharma or to any organization. Rather my allegiance is to my patients and determining the most effective, safest, evidence-based treatments. I strongly feel the standard of care for menopause management needs to be improved.

HOW MY METHOD DIFFERS FROM THE CURRENT "STANDARD OF CARE" MENOPAUSE TREATMENT

Pharmaceutical Topical Estradiol and Pharmaceutical Topical Oral or Vaginal Progesterone

Although topical estradiol is not without risk, a myriad of clinical studies over the last 25 years demonstrate the improved safety of topical estradiol over oral estrogen. Because of fewer risks from topical estradiol, I see no indication for prescribing ORAL estrogen or estrogen injections for chronic therapy. Bioidentical hormones are hormones that are molecularly identical to those present in a woman's body: estradiol, progesterone and testosterone, and are preferred to synthetic hormones. Bioidentical hormones are made by both pharmaceutical companies and compounding pharmacists. Compounding pharmacists mix up various oral and topical preparations in their stores using techniques they learned in pharmacy school. Pharmaceutical companies must meet stricter standards for quality control and efficacy and should be the first therapy of choice over compounded hormones. Topical compounded progesterone has the poorest absorption and should not be used.

Progesterone reduces a woman's risk of uterine cancer. Uterine cancer has been reported from inadequate dosing of topical progesterone.

Monitors Estradiol and Testosterone Blood Tests

Estrogen and testosterone, like other hormones such as thyroid, need to be measured and monitored with blood tests to ensure the lowest therapeutic level that relieves symptoms. The normal pattern of estradiol, progesterone and testosterone seen in the human menstrual cycle was first described in 1971 by Dr. Daniel R. Mishell Jr. These levels guide us in determining optimal dosage of hormones so that therapeutic levels are kept within a physiologic range.

All women are different and variability of absorption has been reported from topical estradiol therapy. Since some women exhibit few symptoms, measuring estradiol levels in patients at risk for serious degenerative diseases such as heart disease, Alzheimer's disease and osteoporosis, ensures therapeutic protective levels. The notion of dosing estrogen in women by "how they feel" is archaic and needs to be brought to the current standards of other endocrine hormone medications. Hopefully, in the future, more dose-response studies will be done to establish optimal therapeutic estradiol blood levels which prevent disease. For the time being, achieving levels at the low end of the physiologic reference range is a prudent course.

Utilizes Cyclic Progesterone Over Daily Progesterone Whenever Possible

In women with an intact uterus, estrogen therapy must be accompanied by appropriate progesterone to protect against an increased risk of uterine cancer that occurs from giving estrogen alone. While continuous progestin protects against uterine cancer, continuous synthetic progestin, as was used in the 2002 Women's Health Initiative (WHI), more often contributes to an increased risk of breast cancer, heart attacks and strokes - hence the reason for recommending progesterone over a synthetic progestin. Giving cyclic progesterone over continuous progesterone comes closer to mimicking the normal physiology of the body.

Replaces Testosterone When Levels Are Deficient

Testosterone plays an important role in modulating the effects of estradiol and can contribute to libido and muscle tone. Some menopausal women continue to produce testosterone from the ovaries or adrenal glands. That's why it is important to measure testosterone blood levels and only provide testosterone replacement if levels are deficient.

Monitors Estrogen Metabolites

Some of the beneficial actions of estradiol occur through its conversion in the liver to certain metabolites or byproducts called "good estrogens." Other liver byproducts of estradiol go through different pathways to produce "bad estrogen" byproducts associated with an increased risk of breast, ovarian and cervical cancers.These estrogen byproducts can all be measured in the urine.

In 2006, a review article in the *New England Journal of Medicine* gave an extensive review of the literature supporting the role of bad estrogen metabolites as cancer initiators. While this may not be the only cause of these cancers, it is a risk factor that can often be modified with healthy lifestyle and supplements. While there are many clinical studies showing benefit, no large randomized, placebo-controlled trials have been done. Clinical research is very costly and since many of these products are non-prescription, there is no financial incentive for companies to fund such research. However, if the therapy is low-risk, why would we NOT want to consider reducing these cancer-promoting byproducts to improve the safety of estrogen therapy?

In addition, recent studies in the cardiology literature show a beneficial byproduct of estradiol produced in the liver that protects against heart disease and also has anti-cancer effects. When deficient, this beneficial byproduct can often be increased by use of supplements. Why would we NOT want to optimize the production of this beneficial byproduct and maximize the benefit of estradiol therapy?

Addresses Postmenopausal Women's Increased Risk for Heart Disease & Strokes

A healthy diet, exercise, and estrogen can lessen the risk of heart disease and strokes, but because of aging, women are still at risk for these diseases. With genetic testing we can identify those at highest risk. Many pharmaceutical medications can provide additional protection and high-risk women should have access to these life-saving therapies.

Because heart disease and strokes occur more commonly in men than women, women are often overlooked in being assessed for these diseases. In 2006, 398,525 American women died of heart attacks and strokes. Compare this to 40,821 women who died of breast cancer that same year. I want to provide women the many benefits of bioidentical hormones and a healthy lifestyle but I don't want to them to die prematurely from heart disease that could have been prevented with pharmaceutical therapy.

Provides Ongoing Monitoring

1. Estradiol blood tests to ensure levels at the lower physiologic range
2. Testosterone blood tests for women receiving testosterone therapy
3. Monitoring advanced lipid and other endocrine and metabolic levels

4. Annual physical exams to assess progress
5. Frequent follow-up visits especially with initiation of estrogen to establish optimal dosage and to monitor other drug therapy
6. Pelvic Exams to monitor for cervical cancer
7. Transvaginal sonograms done yearly to monitor for uterine cancer
8. Mammograms to screen for breast cancer
9. Genetic Counseling and BRCA 1 and BRCA 2 testing for high-risk women as advised by the National Cancer Institute
10. Bone mineral density testing (DEXA) every two years when clinically indicated to check for osteoporosis
11. Carotid intima media thickness test (CIMT) to screen for risk of heart disease and stroke as recommended by the American Heart Association and the American College of Cardiology. CIMT evaluates how well your arteries are aging compared to other women your age. The good news is that it identifies disease in the early stage often before an individual has symptoms and disease can often be improved with the right therapies. Annual CIMTs serve as a parameter to monitor progress

Patient Education

In a managed-care setting, many busy clinicians don't have the time to provide adequate patient education to a postmenopausal woman. Yet in the management of any chronic disease, adequate education and active participation of the patient is essential to their compliance and successful implementation of their program. For example, in diabetes, ancillary staff trained as diabetes educators are essential to optimal management. If physicians don't have time, ancillary staff should be trained to provide this important service.

Summary

Women need to know that ALL estrogens carry risks but the risks are LESS with topical estradiol than with oral or other synthetic estrogens. Importantly, women need to also be informed of the risks of NOT taking estrogen. Many women are routinely medicated with multiple prescription drugs for symptoms that could be easily relieved with an optimal dose of estrogen. Doesn't it make more sense to correct the root cause of the symptom? Such drugs can often be tapered or discontinued resulting in fewer medication risks and cost savings for patients. An educated, informed woman becomes a powerful ally and is more likely to adhere to ongoing treatment, especially when she experiences positive improvements.

As you read through the book you will see how I arrived at this method. Learning and understanding your body is fascinating and will give you a greater understanding of the miracle that is the human body. I challenge you to arm yourself with information so that you can work with your physician and become an active participant in your health.

About the Cover

"Outliving Your Ovaries" Cover Artwork

A special thanks to Maria Rendon, a very talented, award-winning artist from Santa Barbara, California, who provided the design for my book cover. She listened carefully to my philosophy about the importance of treating the whole woman and created a multi-dimensional artwork that enjoys a prominent place in my medical office. Each element represents an integral part of good health and I would like to give you my interpretation of her work.

The figure of a woman arising from the fertile, green earth shows our connection with the cycle of life. All living things are made of organic matter and we all share similar building blocks. Since the reproductive hormones define the essence of woman, the reproductive organs are prominently displayed in a vibrant color resembling blood. The uterus and ovaries are connected to a large, golden treble clef depicting the rest of the endocrine system, an incredibly complex hormone network, akin to a symphony orchestra.

In the center of the chest is a large, golden flower representing the heart, ever beating to drive the life force flowing throughout our bodies. The heart is the seat of the soul and for me, represents my reverence for honoring life. The smaller, flame flowers coming from the woman's hands are her life force being directed externally showing the importance of our relationships to nature and others around us. The blue skies and clouds in her chest depict the healing that comes from breathing in clean, clear air delivering oxygen vital to life. The dark hair studded with stars and the moon represents sleep, another essential healer.

The closed mouth represents the importance of slowing down and attentively listening to the world around you. As a medical student at UCLA, I recall one of my professors telling me, "The patient will always give you the diagnosis, if you just carefully listen to her story." The raindrops surrounding the woman represent water, another healer required by every living organism. Water, the universal solvent, is required by every tissue in our bodies and makes up 55-60% of our bodies. I'll close my impressions of Maria's art with a favorite quote.

> *"An authentically empowered person is humble. This does not mean the false humility of one who stoops to be with those who are below him or her. It is the inclusiveness of one who responds to the beauty of each soul. It is the harmlessness of one who treasures, honors, and reveres life in all its forms."*

> ~ Gary Zukav ~

Me & HRT

Chapter 1

How to read this book

I struggled with providing all the data while not overwhelming the reader with too much technical medical jargon. Since many of you will ultimately be taking this book to your own physician, I wanted the science available so your physician can see it is based on sound medical data. My goal is to provide you and your physician with evidence-based data from the literature. For a lay person, understanding the different types of studies can be confusing.

In general, the "gold standard" in terms of reliability is the *double-blind, placebo-controlled randomized study.* It is often referred to as a randomized, controlled trial or RCT. A placebo is a sugar pill which is given in place of the real medication. Clinical trials show that 30-40% of people may show improvement when given a placebo because they *believe* it will work. In RCTs, a group of individuals on placebo is compared to a group receiving the test medication. In a "double-blind" study neither the study participants nor the researchers know who is getting the real medication. RCTs are also the most expensive type of study and are generally done only after many smaller clinical studies show a possible effect.

An *observational study* is a type of study in which individuals are observed or certain outcomes are measured and no attempt is made to affect the outcome. An *epidemiologic study* compares two groups of people who are alike except for one factor, for example comparing a group of smokers to nonsmokers to evaluate differences in the occurrence of lung cancer. A *meta-analysis* combines results from multiple independent studies of the same problem to increase the statistical power of the analysis. A *prospective cohort* is a type of observational study in which similar individuals (e.g. menopausal women of a certain age) are followed for a number of years to determine the effects of different medications or lifestyle habits on various risks. Whenever possible, I have pointed out the different types of studies.

Some of you may have a science background and be seeking a deeper understanding. For such women, I have provided basic physiology lessons on the most important female hormones, estradiol, progesterone, and testosterone to provide a background for understanding why restoring these hormones is so important to a woman.

Many terms are used for female hormone therapy and there seems to be little consensus since different organizations use different terms! American Association of Clinical Endocrinologists uses hormone replacement therapy (HRT); Endocrine Society uses menopausal hormone therapy (MHT); North American Menopause Society and the American College of Obstetrics & Gynecology uses hormone therapy (HT). The most common term used by the lay public is *hormone replacement therapy* or *HRT.* **Since this book is written for women, I have designated HRT as the term to be used in this book.**

Throughout this book, the term "bioidentical" or "natural" hormone replacement refers to pharmaceutical bioidentical hormone replacement. All published studies on transdermal estradiol have utilized pharmaceutical (NOT compounded) bioidentical hormones.

I have indicated chapters of a more **technical** nature by placing next to the chapter title, a graphic of an atom *(indicating complex details)* in case you want to gloss over that science section or review it at a later time.

I have laid out my philosophical approach to medicine which colors the way I currently treat my patients and why I came to be so passionate about women's health. I have outlined the stages of a woman's reproductive life from the first menstrual period to the last period, the signs and symptoms of menopause, the pros and cons of estrogen replacement and my approach to bioidentical HRT. The *Afterward* brings you full circle and helps the reader understand how we all fit into the circle of life and our connection with Nature.

For those of you who prefer a "Cliff's Notes" approach, you can simply go to the chapters that refer to your stage of life or to those chapters that address your particular questions or concerns.

Many of my patients have kindly reviewed my manuscript and given me very helpful suggestions to make it more patient-friendly. An often repeated comment was, *"I wish I had known about this when I was younger. I would have made different choices if I had known I had other options."* That's why I have added the section on younger women in Chapter 10, *The Reproductive Years.*

Women are often intimidated by the health care system, especially young women in their twenties and thirties. They may suffer needlessly with problem periods or premenstrual syndrome symptoms. When they seek help, birth control pills are often the only treatment offered. I contend the patient is better served when symptoms are relieved by correcting the root cause of the problem.

My goal is to empower women of all ages to have a better understanding of their bodies so they can make more informed choices. Many individuals take better care of their automobiles and their computers than they do of their bodies. Since our bodies do not come with an owner's manual, learning this information can contribute to improved health and vitality for all women.

Chapter 2

As an endocrinologist, I have cared for pre-, peri- and post-menopausal women since 1983. I have written this book because I wanted to give you information about hormone replacement therapy that can have a major impact on your life and health. I also want to share with you how I came to focus on treating menopause. Since 1983, I have personally managed over 100,000 visits with female patients. While there are common patterns, each patient is unique and provides an opportunity to learn another nuance that enriches my understanding of the complexity of the human body.

Practicing clinicians are at the forefront of health care delivery. We first see the unusual patients that don't fit the textbook cases we were taught in medical school. Over the years, I've listened to many menopausal women, carefully monitored their estradiol blood levels, seen what therapies work and which ones don't. Clinical practice is an interplay of listening to the patient, correlating objective tests with symptoms and keeping abreast of the medical literature. When a new study is published that calls for changes in therapy, you make adjustments. It's a dynamic process that requires ongoing "fine-tuning" - that's why it's called the practice of medicine. While I have always held to the principles of bioidentical hormone replacement therapy and monitoring blood hormones, as my knowledge base grows, I continually update my therapies. Much of what drives clinicians are perplexing patients who desperately need our help; it motivates us to be creative at finding solutions.

As a medical student at UCLA, I had the good fortune to be mentored by professors who pioneered the research showing fewer side effects from transdermal estradiol over oral estrogen. Transdermal or dermal is the medical term for delivery of medication applied topically to the skin. However, since this book is directed to the lay public, I have used the term topical throughout the book to make it more understandable for women not familiar with medical jargon. From the time I entered private practice in 1985, I solely utilized topical estradiol. From my training as an endocrinologist and pharmacist, I learned it was prudent and rational to utilize blood estradiol levels to monitor adequacy of dosage. Combining this science-based perspective with my respect for the human body made me a strong proponent of bioidentical hormones. Mother Nature makes fewer mistakes than Man. Doesn't it make more sense to replace the identical deficient hormones instead of confusing the body with synthetic, "wannabe" hormone drugs?

Another issue adding to the confusion of hormone replacement therapy (HRT) for women is the term, "bioidentical hormone replacement therapy." Bioidentical hormones essentially represent those hormones which are molecularly identical to those hormones present in a woman's body: estradiol, progesterone and testosterone. Bioidentical HRT is available from pharmaceutical companies or from compounding pharmacists. Compounding pharmacists are pharmacists who actually mix up the various oral and topical preparations in their stores using techniques they learned in pharmacy school. Pharmacy, like medicine, is a noble profession which has been in existence for centuries. Compounding pharmacists provide a valuable service for patients allergic to pharmaceutical medications or for products that are not commercially available. However, since pharmaceutical bioidentical HRT is readily available and a better product, it should be utilized over compounded HRT.

Bioidentical HRT has developed a very negative connotation because of "turf" battles between pharmaceutical companies and compounding pharmacists. Pharmaceutical companies contend that compounded products don't meet their stricter standards for manufacture and quality control and these are valid considerations. Because compounding pharmacists often don't attach the same warnings that accompany pharmaceutical products, consumers mistakenly think there are no risks to compounded products. The loudest criticism comes from powerful pharmaceutical companies making synthetic oral estrogens that dominate 85% of the market share of estrogen therapy, a $1.3 billion annual market.

In comparison to the pharmaceutical giants making oral, synthetic estrogens, smaller pharmaceutical companies making topical bioidentical hormones are drowned out in the controversy. With such confusion, most women are surprised to learn that bioidentical hormones are readily available from pharmaceutical companies. With such jockeying for market share between competing parties, it's easy to lose sight of the most important issue: what is the best therapy currently available for our patients based on the published medical literature? Truth is the ultimate vector that should drive change and we must recognize our most important priority - the best care of our patients.

It's understandable that companies are driven to protect their financial interests. However, as a practicing physician, I have no vested interest in any of these economic considerations. I don't receive grant funds from any pharmaceutical company. Neither I, nor my family, own any stock in pharmaceutical companies that make HRT. As an advocate for my patients, my role is to select the best therapy for my patients based on the published literature and my clinical experience of 29 years.

This is a primer to enable a woman to read the facts for herself and then discuss it with her own physician to determine what's best for her. I am gratified by the care I've given my patients and those I'll see in the future. However, at this point in my career, I would like to not just see more patients but rather, impart my knowledge and experience to benefit more women.

When I see a woman in menopause, my ultimate job is to prescribe a personalized course of action to help each woman move as successfully as possible through this very difficult and stressful phase of life. Often, the women I see for the first time are deeply troubled by their situation - sometimes desperate for answers and insights. The changes they experience are significant and unsettling, affecting not only them, but others around them as well.

We, of course, need to address their troublesome symptoms. However, what we now know is that there is a window of opportunity lasting just seven to ten years in which women need to make important decisions about whether to take hormones. There are adverse consequences as the years go by without estrogen. As her physician, I work with each woman to guide her toward a course of action that promotes the best outcome for her long-term health.

An endocrinologist specializes in treating disorders of the endocrine system that are usually associated with either deficiency or excess of a particular hormone. The most common diseases managed by endocrinologists are diabetes and hypothyroidism. Endocrinologists with an interest in menopause specialize in helping women understand and manage the effects of menopause. When I was a managed care-physician, like most physicians, I averaged seeing 30 patients a day.

For the past 10 years my practice has transitioned to where I now see four to six patients a day. I have made this conscious decision so I can invest the time necessary to carefully understand and counsel each person who comes to me for care.

I continue to have a deep thirst for knowledge. I'm a voracious reader always looking for opportunities to learn and become a better problem solver and practitioner. I keep an open mind to new and different approaches and stay informed on work being done inside and outside mainstream medicine.

I belong to the American Association of Clinical Endocrinologists (AACE), the Endocrine Society, the North American Menopause Society and the International Society for the Study of Women's Sexual Health. I'm also a member of the Institute for Functional Medicine (IFM). This latter group is vital in my study of preventive medicine and the pursuit of natural approaches to healing. My Texas medical license requires 12.5 hours per year of continuing medical education (CME), but I average about 60+ hours. Medicine is ever changing. I attend CME conferences held by all these organizations to stay current on issues and findings relevant to my practice.

I admire the philosophy of one of the 16th century founders of medicine, *Paracelsus*. He believed the health of the body relied on the harmony of man, the microcosm, with Nature, the macrocosm. *Paracelsus* made a sojourn to many cultures eager to learn new therapies that could benefit his patients. To me it's just common sense - why would I not want to know about any therapy that might expand my understanding and benefit my patients? My patients love the fact that I give them the best of both worlds - traditional medicine and natural medicine. So often one group never communicates with the other and patient care suffers.

An essential aspect of my learning comes from my daily inter-
actions with my patients. I acquired important clinical skills
in medical school, but it is from my patients that I learned
about life. As I listen to my patients' stories, I am in awe of
the power of the human spirit and its capacity to overcome
adversity. I'm inspired by my patients' trust and faith in a
power beyond themselves. They are my rock and define
who I am. I feel very privileged to have been entrusted with
their care and I so want to help them. Seeking solutions to
their problems gives me the motivation to keep learning and
growing.

I often describe myself as a medical *Sherlock Holmes*. Determining the underlying cause of patients' signs and symptoms
enables me to develop plans of action that alleviate their
symptoms. I help them see why they got ill and understand
the process we must follow to regain their health. In this way,
my patients and I become a formidable team working toward
the common goal of their optimal health. It's incredibly gratifying to see the delight in their eyes when they truly compre-
hend the process and experience the results. While women
make up the majority of my practice, I continue to treat
general endocrine problems and often see men as well. I have
a lot of "couple patients." Quite often, whichever spouse sees
me first will eventually introduce his or her partner, wanting
the other to experience optimal health as well.

I've found that people are often confused by the hierarchy of
medicine. All physicians can be categorized either as a medical
specialty or a surgical specialty. All are essential to the health
care system but their training and perspective are markedly different. Although endocrinologists are the hormone specialists,
most women's hormones are actually prescribed by gynecologists. A primary reason for this is that there are many more

ob/gyn's than endocrinologists. A woman rightfully develops a trusting relationship with her ob/gyn, especially the one who delivered her babies. However, a basic difference between a gynecologist and an endocrinologist is that the ob/gyn is trained as a surgeon and the endocrinologist is an internist - each approaches problems from a very different mind-set.

Endocrinologists must first complete a three year residency in internal medicine. Then they undergo specialty training in endocrinology for two to three additional years. Endocrinologists/internists are trained to determine the underlying disease process - to treat it medically and whenever possible, to reduce or prevent the need for surgery. Whenever a patient fails medical therapy, I often require the expertise of a gynecologist to perform a procedure or surgery.

Often times to a surgeon, "to cut is to cure." Of course, gynecologists have to have good justification to perform surgery and they have a totally different skill set that endocrinologists cannot provide. Most women are seen by ob-gyn's only once a year for their pelvic exam. A woman may develop heavy bleeding in the interim between visits and by the time she comes back for her yearly visit, her bleeding may have worsened to the point that surgery is required. But if you strive to understand your body, become accountable and take responsibility for your health, you might be able to avoid surgery. Learning the subtle changes that occur in perimenopause and menopause can prompt you to see your physician sooner, whether he/she is a gynecologist, internist, family practitioner or endocrinologist. A better understanding of your body enables you to convey important symptoms, ask the right questions and better evaluate the treatment plan offered by your physician. Your proactive behavior can often prevent your need to undergo a hysterectomy. I hope to give you information and guidance to help you have a better dialogue with your physician.

Women who become my patients often ask me, *"Why didn't my gynecologist give me these hormones?"* To this I tell them, physicians are overwhelmed with a plethora of medical literature that comes out each and every day. It is unfair to expect that an ob/gyn can keep up with ALL the surgical and medical literature in obstetrics, gynecology, endocrinology and internal medicine. I certainly don't have a wide knowledge base in obstetrics and surgical gynecology. The same concept applies to family practice physicians who have an even broader scope of practice. Patients need to understand that each specialty has value and has developed because it is necessary to provide comprehensive care.

All physicians want the best for our patients. If you become informed and discuss with them a plan for hormone replacement that has scientific basis in the medical literature, your physician is likely to be amenable to prescribing such a program. However, it's not "one size fits all" and ultimately any hormone replacement therapy (HRT) protocol needs to be fine-tuned to accommodate your particular needs. For example, when prescribing thyroid medications for a patient, physicians may carefully decide between minute doses, i.e. should we give 0.112 or 0.125 mg of levothyroxine? This same principle of determining optimal dosage should be applied to developing a personalized hormone regimen for each woman.

In my practice, I seek to understand the patient on a human level as well as on a molecular level. When I design a therapeutic and preventive program for a patient, my goal is to first support the intrinsic, healing mechanisms of the body, to replace deficient hormones and to restore dysfunctional systems to an optimal state. In this manner, the patient and physician are working with the body to engage its enormous capacity for self-healing.

When I became an endocrinologist, I made sure that my mother's physician prescribed hormone therapy throughout her post-menopausal years. She had such a zest for living and maintaining her independence. She never once hesitated about taking hormones or complained about the frequent blood tests I ordered to keep her finely tuned. At 84, she still lived in her own home, did her own cooking, and loved to read. She always went for her 30-minute walk, rain or shine. She was a role model for me of how to live and enjoy your older years.

I believe we have a responsibility not only to ourselves, but also to our families and society, to maintain our health and productivity for as long as possible. Baby Boomers, by our sheer numbers, will bankrupt the healthcare system if we don't take charge of our own health. Imagine the cost to the healthcare system when we 76 million Boomers hit 80 years of age. It has been estimated that 30% of Medicare dollars are spent in keeping patients alive in the last four weeks of their life. Contrast that with the enormous potential savings to society if we each take preventive medical measures that enable us to not only enjoy our independence, but to also compress those pre-terminal health costs to a few days instead of several years.

I love listening to my patients, hearing their stories and learning the many nuances of expression of various diseases. This is the art and joy of medicine: applying general medical knowledge to that individual patient so we can provide more personalized care. Patients can better relate to complex medical material when they hear examples that apply to them. So I am sharing some of my patients' stories throughout this book but I've taken extra care to safeguard their privacy. I have also added a few personal notes and observations that reflect my wonder when I contemplate the miracle of the human body. I see the body-mind of man and of woman as a work of art and as perfection in form and function. Human life is a treasure and I'd like for this book to help you safeguard that treasure.

I believe you'll find great value in this book. It is not intended to be an encyclopedia on menopause. Rather it is a guide to help you understand the risks and benefits of hormone replacement therapy. Arming yourself with this knowledge enables you to better participate with your physician in deciding the best course of action for you.

Marina Johnson, M.D., F.A.C.E
Medical Director
Board Certified in Endocrinology and Internal Medicine
The Institute of Endocrinology and Preventive Medicine

Chapter 3

*Improving patient outcomes
in chronic disease*

I believe our health care system needs to be more patient-centered and engage patients in their own care. American medicine excels at crisis intervention with innovative drugs and surgical procedures. Yet chronic illness comprises the majority of problems that most physicians see in their office. Chronic health problems are adversely affected by poor diet, lack of exercise, obesity, smoking and excess alcohol. Another factor affecting chronic disease management is that insurance companies typically do not reimburse for measures to prevent disease. They instead wait until a serious disease has occurred that generally is much more costly to treat.

In a commentary published in the *Journal of the American Medical Association* 2004, Dr. Halsted Holman from Stanford Medical School addressed the fact that medical schools have not adequately prepared new physicians for managing chronic illness and acknowledged that changes need to be made in the curriculum to deal with this important health issue. Patients with chronic illness who lack understanding of their disease are less likely to comply with the lifestyle changes necessary to enhance the physician's therapy.

Integrative medicine is a more inclusive approach to managing chronic illness. Several exemplary medical schools like *UCLA, Harvard, Stanford* and *UC San Francisco (UCSF)* have established centers for integrative medicine. There are currently 40 integrative medicine fellowship programs at medical schools in the United States.

UCSF was the first integrative medicine center established in 1996 and defines integrative medicine in the following way:

> *"Integrative medicine is a new term that emphasizes the combination of both conventional and alternative approaches to address the biological, psychological, social and spiritual aspects of health and illness. It emphasizes respect for the human capacity for healing, the importance of the relationship between the physician and the patient, a collaborative approach to patient care among practitioners, and the practice of conventional, complementary and alternative health care that is evidence-based."*

Functional medicine is the next evolution of integrative medicine that incorporates all the conventional and alternative evidence-based options within an informational framework that enables you to detect the intrinsic mechanisms that may be driving the problem. The model is based on a systems biology perspective in which the interconnectedness of all the body systems is taken into consideration. All of our body organs and systems talk to each other and dysfunction in one system can result in disease in other parts of the body. It's not exclusive or inclusive of any particular treatment modality or test, so surgery could be functional medicine. Recognizing and treating the underlying cause of symptoms enables the physician to engage the body's capacity for self-healing.

Learning To Think Outside the Box

As a new physician, I thought I "knew it all." However, I quickly learned in those first few years that medical school simply gives you the tools with which to evaluate the thousands of different patients you'll see in your career. Even with those great tools, you must pursue ongoing medical education or you quickly become outdated. It's definitely a stressful life, but gratifying when you find answers and relieve suffering. When faced with a sick patient for whom standard treatments are not working, physicians feel compelled to look for other options to relieve that patient's suffering.

I saw such a patient in the 1990's who caused my practice to take a turn in the road. I had a very busy managed care practice at that time. I had acquired a reputation among my colleagues as someone who was a very good diagnostician. Jane was a very pleasant patient sent to me by her family doctor. She complained of generalized symptoms of severe fatigue, poor concentration, irritability and joint pains which were making it difficult to care for herself and her family. She had been given pain pills for the joint pains that only made her fatigue and poor concentration worse. She told me her doctor said, *"I don't know what you have, but I want you to go see Dr. Johnson. If she can't help you, then you'll need to go see a shrink!"* I did an endocrine evaluation and her test results all came back normal. I felt very badly for her because I knew she wasn't "making up the symptoms" but yet I had no idea what was going on with her or what to do to help her.

I could have referred her back to her doctor saying I didn't see an endocrine problem. However, I knew that if I did that she would just be prescribed an array of psychotropic drugs. In no way am I disparaging the important role that psychiatrists play in managing psychiatric patients. It's just that sometimes in a busy practice, when the medical physician doesn't know what's going on with a particular patient, there's a tendency to write the patient off as being "crazy." In my opinion, this patient had neither a psychiatric nor an endocrine problem but I didn't know what to do for her or where to send her. I wanted so much to help her that I had to start thinking more creatively.

It turned out while Jane did not have an endocrine problem, she did have a very significant, digestive problem and was having frequent, loose bowel movements each day. She had previously seen a gastroenterologist who had done a colonoscopy and told her everything was normal. He diagnosed her with irritable bowel syndrome (IBS). IBS is a "catch all" phrase given to patients after serious pathology has been excluded. Gastroenterologists tend to focus on treating seriously ill patients with colon cancer, bleeding ulcers and other digestive conditions that often require hospitalization. Since IBS is regarded as a chronic, benign condition, such patients are generally referred back to their general practitioner. Because patients are reassured by the benign colonoscopy, they may resign themselves and think these symptoms are "normal" for them. This often occurs, especially with digestive problems because many people are embarrassed to discuss their bowel habits with friends or family so they don't know what constitutes normal bowel habits.

Since every endocrinologist is first trained in internal medicine, I did have training in digestive disorders in my residency program. However, it wasn't until I studied integrative medicine and functional medicine that I became aware of the importance of the gastrointestinal (GI) tract to good health.

The GI tract contains 60% of your immune system and produces 90% of your serotonin, the feel-good neurotransmitter which contributes to energy, good sleep and a sense of well-being. I did diagnostic tests and determined she had an intestinal bacterial infection causing her IBS. Once her infection was treated with an antibiotic, she had resolution of her loose stools. The GI tract is essential for absorption of nutrients that serve as building blocks to repair cells and make new ones. After restoring normal GI function, all her symptoms resolved and both of us were delighted with her recovery!

Chapter 4

Principles influencing
my approach to medicine

Solutions Not Suppression™

I'm a naturally curious person which greatly affects how
I evaluate a patient. I see signs and symptoms as the language
of the body. This is how your body tells you and me there is a
problem. Symptoms represent a reactive compensation of the
body to an underlying process. Once I understand the process
that caused the symptoms, I'm in a better position to formu-
late a plan to correct the problem.

When physicians don't truly understand the nature of a
disease, they'll often describe it and then add "syndrome"
to the end. For example, the cause of Chronic Fatigue Syndrome is not known but there is a typical clinical picture.
By giving it a label, everyone understands what we're
describing. This is also the way insurance companies
categorize patients to determine payment for physician
services. This process can be useful but it is also problematic
when the patients become merely labels and all therapy is
aimed at simply treating superficial symptoms. For example,
giving amphetamines to a patient with chronic fatigue may
give them short-term relief but it is rarely a long-term solution and does not address the cause of the symptom.

Betty, a school teacher in her thirties, had an obvious tremor
in both hands. She was an attractive, young woman but she

was sitting there with a fine tremor that got worse when she tried to do anything with her hands. She had difficulty holding a coffee cup or even writing a check so you can imagine how disabling it would be for a teacher who has to write on the blackboard and grade homework. I was very concerned that someone so young would be having such symptoms. Therefore, I ordered a number of tests to try to determine if there was some underlying disease or unknown exposure to toxins that could be damaging her nervous system. The patient didn't return for a follow-up so we called to inquire about her. She said she'd gone to another physician who diagnosed her immediately on her very first visit. I eagerly asked what he had diagnosed. With great pleasure, she announced, *"I have Essential Tremors Syndrome and I was given a medicine (anti-seizure medicine) that made it go away."* I worried that taking this medicine for years would delay discovery of the underlying process causing the tremors.

I was also concerned because chronic medication use can result in adverse effects. Adverse effects from chronic medications may not show up for years. Most people don't know that when a new drug is released, it has usually only been tested in a few thousand people for less than three months. It isn't until the drug has been used in millions of patients for many years that the serious side effects become apparent. Phen/Fen and Vioxx should be keen reminders to us all. However, Betty didn't want to hear any of this discussion. She had been given a "diagnosis" that completely satisfied her. All I could do was wish her well.

To me, the endocrinologist is akin to a systems analyst for the body. The body is a highly complex system of interlinked processes constantly changing within a delicate balance called homeostasis. Signs and symptoms often indicate underlying disturbances in that balance so when you correct the under-lying problem, you resolve the symptoms. Giving a pill that simply masks the symptom is like "killing the messenger." I prefer to relieve the symptoms by correcting the underly-ing process that causes the symptom. Many patients who see me are searching for these kinds of answers. For example, deficiency in thyroid hormone can cause many symptoms including fatigue, dry skin, hair loss, constipation, depression and weight gain. Each symptom can be treated by a myriad of medications each of which carries side effects. However, most of these symptoms are relieved with the right dose of thyroid hormone. What could be more elegant?

The Risk-Benefit Ratio

This bias in my practice stems from my pharmacist training which taught me to always carefully consider the risk-benefit ratio of any therapy. My knowledge of pharmacology gives me a healthy respect for pharmaceutical drugs. They can be marvelous, life-saving medications but some can have toxic side effects. I have a very practical approach to selecting therapies for my patients. If a problem can be treated with diet and exercise, that's my first choice. If these are not adequate and it's a mild condition, I'll replace deficient vita-mins or minerals and occasional herbal therapy. If none of these measures work, I'll select a pharmaceutical drug - but even then I'll always consider the safety profile of that drug. You don't use an elephant gun to kill a mosquito. Conversely, if a person has a serious condition like a heart attack, I'm not going to solely treat them with vitamins. A physician must always temper therapy to the severity of the problem. So, I use caution in prescribing toxic drugs for the treatment of mild chronic problems that can be addressed with safer, nonpre-scription, therapy.

My Role as a Patient Advocate

When patients select me to be their physician, I have an ethical responsibility to choose the best and safest course of therapy for their particular situation. This filter colors every aspect of my practice. Because I am their advocate, patients often ask my advice about elective surgeries or assistance in helping them select the most skilled surgeon.

I wanted to become knowledgeable about nutritional and herbal therapies among others, because my patients needed guidance in selecting the best therapies from the overwhelming numbers available to them. Who better to advise them than their own physician who knows their particular health problems and needs?

I prescribe bioidentical HRT because, in my clinical experience and from my continuing review of the literature, they are a safer choice for my patients. Bioidentical HRT involves the use of medications that are identical in chemical structure to those hormones present in your body. It carries risks like any prescription medicine, and women need to be informed of those risks. Patients are usually surprised to learn that bioidentical hormones are easily available from pharmaceutical companies. I have used compounded hormones in special circumstances but the majority of my therapy is pharmaceutical bioidentical hormones. The physician must monitor blood levels of both compounded and pharmaceutical products to ensure proper dosage for each patient.

Patient Education and Accountability for Self-Care

In the management of any chronic condition, each patient must have a basic understanding of her health problems so she and her physician can work as a team toward a common goal of improving her health. The physician should explain issues in easy-to-understand lay terms. I love teaching my patients. After all, the Latin meaning for doctor is "teacher," and physicians have a responsibility to teach patients about their bodies. In a busy managed-care setting where a patient spends an average of eight minutes with her physician, women are often left confused about exactly what they are supposed to do and why. Patients tend to comply better when they understand the importance and consequences of their actions. They need to know all their options and participate in decision-making, with their physician's guidance.

In diabetes management, patient education can be critical in preventing kidney failure, blindness, amputations and heart disease. Endocrinologists form teams of trained nurses and dietitians to provide this patient education. I applied similar principles of good diabetes management to menopause management and have found it exceedingly helpful at improving patient outcomes. Any program that I create for a patient necessarily requires that she accept responsibility for complying with the therapy. It greatly improves compliance with medications and making lifestyle changes in diet and exercise. No one is expected to be perfect but being engaged and committed to the plan makes for a better outcome. Individuals who think they can simply take a pill while continuing self-destructive lifestyles experience disappointing results.

Healing begins by knowing that it is possible

Giving patients hope is an important aspect of the doctor-patient relationship that contributes to good outcomes. Early on in my career as a new endocrinologist, I saw Alice, a 35-year-old woman with Type 1 diabetes and mild diabetic kidney damage. I started her on a protein-restricted diet and medication to slow the progression of diabetic kidney disease. Eager to not be missing any other new therapy that might be helpful, I referred her to a kidney specialist. Alice came back to see me two weeks later, and burst into tears as soon as I entered the exam room. Alarmed at her distress, I asked what had happened. Through her tears, she sobbed, *"I went to the nephrologist and showed him all the lab results you had done and your recommendations which he advised me to continue. Then he showed me a graph outlining the progression of diabetic kidney disease. He told me, based on your lab values, this is where you are now and in 4.2 years, you will have end-stage kidney failure and need to start on dialysis!"*

That nephrologist was a fledgling physician, like myself, and he was probably trying to be very scientific in presenting Joni the most precise data. What I learned from that experience was that a physician's words can be destructive or healing. Giving Joni such cold, hard facts implied her progression to kidney failure was inevitable. In any study, there are always "outliers", who do better than the "average" participant. It is important to not give false hopes, but patients should be encouraged to defy the odds because the patient's mental state and perception have a powerful effect on self-healing.

Chapter 5

Why my interest in menopause?

The structure and operation of the human body is intriguing. It is a beautifully linked, complex system involving endless, intricate processes. I am in awe of this system and have dedicated my life to honoring it and understanding it as completely as possible. Even though I had an excellent education at UCLA and USC, I've learned even more over the years by listening to and interacting with my patients. Medicine is a life-long process of learning, continually enhanced as a physician acquires and draws upon a rich knowledge base of clinical experience.

My interest in menopause began as a teenager. In high school in the late 1960s, I recall my friends' mothers in their forties and fifties being hospitalized for "nervous breakdowns." I thought it was curious that so many women were supposedly having nervous breakdowns. Now I realize they were probably going through menopause. Unfortunately, far too often women's complaints are trivialized or dismissed as being hysterical. The Latin word *hystericus*, formed the basis of the modern Latin noun, hysteria, a term coined in the 19th century for a neurotic condition supposedly peculiar to women. This forms the origin of hysterectomy, the medical term for removal of the uterus

When I decided to go to medical school, I swore I would do something to improve health care for women. Even today, when women in their forties complain of depression, mood swings and anxiety, it's common for them to be prescribed antidepressants and tranquilizers before being considered for hormones. To be sure, these medications have an important role, especially in patients with severe symptoms. However, if the symptoms occur in the presence of an underlying deficiency of estrogen, testosterone, or thyroid hormone, it's essential to correct the underlying hormone deficiency.

When I was first starting my medical practice, menopausal problems were not taken very seriously. Hot flashes and premenstrual syndrome (PMS) were the source of a lot of jokes. Well, it isn't funny when you feel awful and your life is falling apart. I can't tell you how many times I've had women apologize for "wasting my time" with their complaints or tell me, *"Thank you for listening to me."* I would always assure them that hearing their symptoms is essential for my finding the correct solution for their problem.

There are a few patients seared into my memory bank who forever changed my attitude about menopause. I once was called to do an endocrine consultation on Joan, a patient in the psychiatric ICU with "hirsutism" or excess facial hair. When I went to see Joan, she indeed had a moderate degree of facial hair. However, after reviewing her chart, I was astonished to learn that she'd been a banker with no prior psychiatric history. She'd undergone a total hysterectomy with removal of her ovaries for a benign condition the summer before and I was horrified to learn that she'd never been given hormone replacement.

After the surgery, her mental condition deteriorated to the point where she'd lost her job. She was put on various psychotropic medications but continued to do poorly. She'd become suicidal and ultimately was admitted to the psychiatric intensive care unit. It had not occurred to anyone that perhaps she needed hormones. When I started her on HRT, I saw firsthand how restoring deficient hormones can produce a total transformation in a person's life. This woman eventually went off all her psychotropic medicines and was able to go back to her normal life. It still brings tears to my eyes as I think about how she was made to suffer needlessly. At the same time, it is incredibly gratifying when you can use your training and experience to help a person become whole again. That's what drives most physicians - the desire to relieve suffering and help people.

Because menopause is something every woman goes through, it's often not even considered a medical problem. Women frequently ask me, *"Isn't it better that I go through menopause naturally? My grandmother lived to be 90 years old and she never took hormones."* To this I say, *"What was the quality of your grandmother's life at 90? Was she in full possession of all her faculties, free of osteoporosis and was she self-sufficient? If she was, then maybe you don't need to take hormones."* My purpose is not to coerce anyone to take hormones but rather to present facts and options to help you make a more informed decision.

In my own dear mother's case, I made sure she was prescribed estrogen by her gynecologist. At age 84, she still lived in her own home, did her own cooking and cared for my 91-year-old father. She walked two miles every day, had an active mind and loved books, garage sales and visiting with her friends. They'd ask her, *"How do you keep so active? What's your secret?"* She'd smile proudly and say, *"My daughter, the doctor, takes good care of me."* One Friday she went for her usual walk, went to two garage sales and had lunch with her best friend. That evening she had the worst headache she had ever had and was admitted to the hospital with a massive stroke. She lingered for three days and quietly died - but only after each of her

five children had arrived to be at her bedside. Our family was
shocked to have our active, vibrant mother die so suddenly,
but in retrospect, we realized we should all be so lucky. That's
how I want to die - happy, independent, living in my own
home and taking care of myself.

Consider this: In the 1800s, many women died during childbirth and it was common for men to have several wives in
succession. In 1900, the average age of menopause was 50
to 55, much as it is today. However, in 1900 the average life
expectancy for women was 50! Today's women have a life expectancy that approaches 80. *We're now routinely outliving our
ovaries. God has granted us 30 extra years of life after menopause. What are we to do with this precious gift?*

Will we squander it by spending three decades suffering the
physical, emotional and mental symptoms of estrogen deficiency? Will you spend the last 10 years vegetating in a nursing home? If you need an incentive to take hormones, look at
the empty faces of women in nursing homes who are simply
waiting to die. I believe we have a responsibility to ourselves
and to our families to remain healthy and productive as long
as possible.

It's been estimated that 6000 women in the U.S. become
menopausal every day. That is four women every minute.
According to the US Census statistics, there were 46 million
women in 2000 and that number is expected to increase to
50 million by the year 2020. Can you imagine the drain on
our health care system if the majority of us Baby Boomers
enter advanced menopause without hormones? It will surely
bankrupt the system and place an unnecessary burden on our
children's economy. I think society will be much better off if
we can follow my mother's example of self-sufficiency.

Helping women in menopause is an opportunity to transform lives and enable women to achieve their full potential. I spend a great deal of time teaching patients how to practice healthy habits that greatly enhance the medical therapy I provide. I believe many of the problems present in our healthcare system today could be improved if people would become more accountable and take more personal responsibility for keeping themselves healthy.

Since becoming an endocrinologist in 1983, I have had over 100,000 patient visits with pre-, peri- and postmenopausal women. I have primarily used topical estradiol since 1986 when the first pharmaceutical estradiol was introduced. I have tried compounded topical estradiol products but have consistently found them less effective and reliable such that now pharmaceutical topical estradiol is always my first choice. My current clinical practice represents an evolving, ever-changing refinement as new studies come out requiring adjustments to my therapies.

Because of my passion to improve women's health, I would like to share with my readers the benefit of my years of clinical experience and help you in understanding the current published studies that have led to my current therapies. I have drawn on my previous work as an assistant editor for a drug publication and I have read over 450 published medical articles to write this book. Because I was a pharmacist before medical school, I can help you understand the political climate that has added to the confusion surrounding HRT.

The Debate Over Hormone Therapy

Fewer than 20 percent of menopausal women in the United States take hormones. Of those women given prescriptions for hormones, half of them discontinue therapy after the first year. If we had a 20 percent compliance rate in treating hypertension, it would be considered an urgent public health issue. Menopause is a deficiency state associated with many health consequences that markedly affect the quality of a woman's life and those around her. Why do women deny themselves the benefits of hormones?

I contend the problem lies with the great confusion among patients and physicians over perceived risks and benefits. Women know hormones relieve menopausal symptoms, but they are faced with conflicting data on the safety of taking hormone replacement therapy (HRT). They are presented the increased risks of taking HRT without considering the risks of NOT taking estrogen. Most American women are given oral hormone regimens or continuous synthetic progestins that carry more side effects than topical therapies. Women are sometimes given "one size fits all" regimens instead of considering their individual needs.

It's important to consider the facts and use common sense. The mass media may sometimes sensationalize news to make it sound more compelling. The decision whether to take HRT is far too important to be based on a few sound bites. It requires careful research and a discussion with your physician about the pros and cons of hormone replacement within the context of your particular circumstance and overall health. This book will provide you data you need to make an informed decision on HRT. I've gathered information from a variety of sources and combined it with all the knowledge I've gained from my experience as a pharmacist, from my years of medical training, from decades of medical practice, and from listening carefully to my patients.

Understanding a Woman's Body

Chapter 6

The symphony within:
The endocrine system

To make the proper choice regarding hormone replacement, it's important to understand the basic function of the endocrine system - that complex and elegant chemical enterprise within the body that controls and coordinates such functions as reproduction, metabolism, behavior, growth and development. Replenishing and rebalancing of this system are the goals of hormone replacement and the focus of endocrinology.

Within the endocrine system, 10 or more major endocrine glands and a number of minor ones secrete hormones, or chemical messengers, that mediate communication between cells. The body seeks to establish a state called homeostasis - *a perfect balance.* It is an elaborate bodily harmony not unlike that created by the instruments of a symphony orchestra. One player out of tune diminishes the performance of the entire orchestra. Like the symphony, the harmonic interplay of the endocrine glands and the hormones they produce creates the beauty and power of the concert.

Hormones are molecules that act as signals from one type of cell to another. Most hormones reach their target cells via the bloodstream. The word itself is from the Greek word *"horman"* meaning "to set in motion" or "to excite." Resuming the analogy of the symphony orchestra, the body has a number of section leaders controlling and regulating the woodwinds, brass, percussion and strings - these are the hormones and hormone-like substances of the endocrine system. The conductor of these control centers is the pituitary, often called the "king of glands." The pituitary is the size and shape of a pea, and it has an intimate connection with the hypothalamus, which is actually part of the brain. More specifically, the hypothalamus is the interface between the brain and the endocrine system. Each gland has a corresponding hormone in the pituitary that regulates the function of that gland. In this manner, all the glands of the endocrine system are ultimately under the control of the brain.

In the following chapters, I will focus on the reproductive system that is largely controlled by the ovaries that produce estradiol, progesterone, and testosterone. The pituitary hormones that regulate the ovaries are called follicle-stimulating hormone (FSH) and luteinizing hormone (LH). The hypothalamus secretes gonadotropin-releasing hormone (GnRH) that turns on the pituitary production of FSH and LH.

However, keep in mind that optimal function of the reproductive system can also be affected by the other hormones of the endocrine symphony.

Diagram of the Female Endocrine System

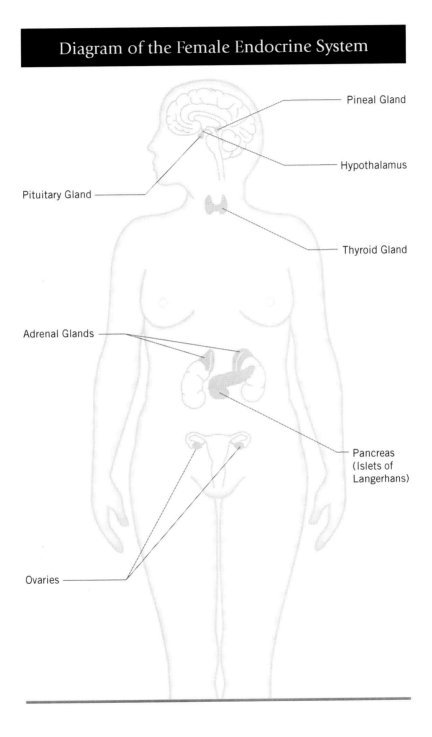

Pineal Gland

Hypothalamus

Pituitary Gland

Thyroid Gland

Adrenal Glands

Pancreas
(Islets of
Langerhans)

Ovaries

Chapter 7

Hormones of the reproductive system

❈

Understanding the biology and physiology of estradiol, progesterone, and testosterone gives us insight on how critical they are to the optimal function of the body. When they are deficient, as in menopause, it's preferable, whenever possible, to utilize bioidentical hormones to restore the very same hormones which have been in your body since you went through puberty. Cholesterol, which some people regard as something "bad", is actually the basic building block for all the hormones made by the ovaries and the adrenal glands. Care should be taken to not aggressively lower cholesterol to extremely low levels with cholesterol lowering drugs because it can cause marked disruption in production of these vital hormones.

Jerry, a 58-year-old successful businessman, came to see me because of fatigue and sexual dysfunction. Because of his fatigue he was considering selling his business and taking early retirement. He had always enjoyed a healthy sex drive and lots of energy but now he was considering "calling it quits" and taking early retirement.

I diagnosed him with profoundly low testosterone but I also noted that his total cholesterol was only 105! I learned he had been started on a cholesterol lowering drug the previous year that corresponded to the time frame when he developed his sexual dysfunction and fatigue. I made a modest reduction in his cholesterol medication and his testosterone level normalized without the need for testosterone replacement.

Cholesterol lowering drugs can be life-saving but all these possible effects need to be considered. All this is further evidence that everything in our body is there for a reason. When you introduce drugs that cause drastic changes, adverse consequences can occur.

Estradiol and its functions

Although estradiol is the principle hormone secreted by the ovary, it actually comes from testosterone and androstenedione. Androstenedione is found in the ovary and fat cells and gets converted to estrone and ultimately to estradiol. Testosterone is also present in the ovary and in fat cells. As you'll learn in a later chapter, the higher testosterone, androstenedione, and estrone in fat cells in obese women explains their increased risk of cancer. Recall that cholesterol is the initial building block for all these hormones. Estriol is a weaker, breakdown byproduct of estrone and estradiol which is produced in the liver.

The typical functions attributed to estrogen include the development of most sexual characteristics in a female and the growth and development of the female sexual organs. Specifically these include the following:

- Stimulating the lining of the uterus to grow
- Regulating the menstrual cycles and reproduction
- Stimulating breast development and maturation
- Maintaining the thickness of the vaginal wall

However, there are many more effects of estrogen beyond the reproductive system that are essential to the health of the body. First, let's talk about hormone receptors so you can understand how these systemic effects were discovered.

Most hormones, including estrogen, do their work by linking up with a receptor. Sometimes receptors are located on the lining of the cell called the cell membrane. Other receptors are located on the nucleus inside the cell. You can think of a hormone and its receptor as a key and lock mechanism. The hormone is the key required to open the lock of the receptor that allows entry of the hormone into the cell or nucleus to do its work.

In the case of estrogen, the estrogen receptor, the lock, is present on the nucleus of the cell. Only estrogen or an estrogen-like substance can interact with that receptor. When estrogen combines with its estrogen receptor, it allows entry of the estrogen into the nucleus. There it combines with various genes and sets in motion a series of instructions that results in the production of various proteins. This action of estrogen is called a genomic effect because it is mediated through action on your genes - the DNA in your cells. You can think of the DNA as the library of genetic instructions that tells your body how to maintain the upkeep of the body. When estrogen acts on the DNA, it produces a substance called messenger RNA that gives instructions to the mitochondria, the factory in the cell where the proteins will be produced. When the nucleus sends out messenger RNA, it's like checking a "how-to" book out of the library.

Estrogen receptors have been discovered on many tissues throughout the body including the brain, lungs, heart, liver, blood vessels, kidney, breast, skin, ovary, uterus, vagina, and bones. The presence of estrogen receptors on so many tissues suggests great importance of estrogen to the optimal function of the entire body. There are two kinds of estrogen receptors: alpha and beta. More is known about the alpha receptor because it was discovered in the 1950's while the beta receptor was only discovered in 1996.

You can think of the alpha and beta receptors of estrogen as representing the yin and yang effects of estradiol. The alpha receptor causes growth of tissue while the beta receptor tones down the action of the alpha by inhibiting excess growth. It's fascinating how the body has such intrinsic protective mechanisms. It has been hypothesized that enhancing the estradiol beta receptor would be another useful way to protect against breast cancer. Women with breast cancer are often treated with aromitase inhibitor drugs that stimulate the beta receptor. There are herbs that preferentially enhance the beta receptor and may be useful in prevention of breast cancer.

In addition to estrogen effects on your DNA - genomic actions - estrogen has additional actions on other tissues called non-genomic effects because they occur without interacting with your genes. The following are actions of estrogen unrelated to sexual function or reproduction.

Actions of Estrogen against heart disease:

1. Protects the blood vessels in the heart and kidneys against forming plaque and inflammation by preventing over-growth of smooth muscle cells and dilating blood vessels
2. Increases production of HDL and decreases LDL
3. Prevents platelets from clotting too quickly and decreases harmful levels of homocysteine

Actions of Estrogen against osteoporosis:

1. Decreasing breakdown of bone
2. Increasing calcium absorption in the digestive system

Actions of Estrogen against Alzheimer's, dementia & loss of cognitive function:

1. Increases cerebral blood flow
2. Protects against apoptosis (programmed cell death)
3. Anti-inflammatory effect on the brain
4. Antioxidant effects which reduce harmful substances called "free radicals"
5. Helps to regulate body temperature
6. Modulates synapses which are the special junctions where nerve cells communicate with each other
7. Stimulates the hippocampus (located near the bottom of the front of the brain) which is important for memory and learning

Progesterone and its functions

Progesterone is produced by the corpus luteum of the ovary during the last half of the menstrual cycle.

Actions of progesterone include the following:

1. Counters the effect of estradiol on the endometrium to prevent excessive growth
2. Prepares the endometrium of the uterus for a potential pregnancy
3. Helps in maintenance of pregnancy
4. Prepares the breasts for lactation
5. Decreases uterine contractions
6. Signals the beginning of labor
7. Functions in the brain to mediate the sexual response
8. Appears to have some benefit on bone

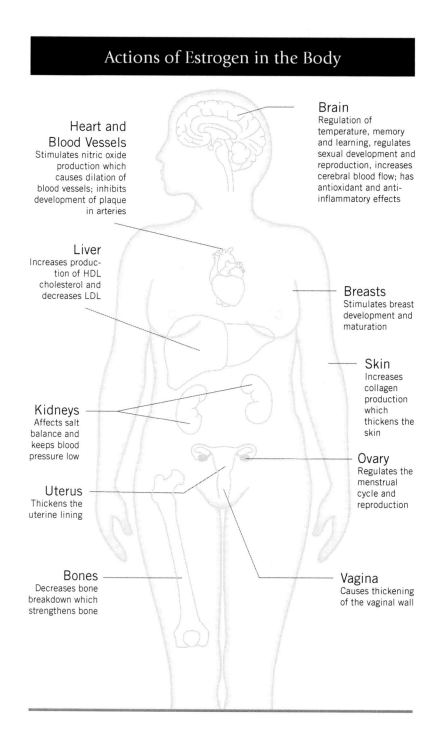

Actions of Estrogen in the Body

Brain
Regulation of temperature, memory and learning, regulates sexual development and reproduction, increases cerebral blood flow; has antioxidant and anti-inflammatory effects

Heart and Blood Vessels
Stimulates nitric oxide production which causes dilation of blood vessels; inhibits development of plaque in arteries

Liver
Increases production of HDL cholesterol and decreases LDL

Breasts
Stimulates breast development and maturation

Skin
Increases collagen production which thickens the skin

Kidneys
Affects salt balance and keeps blood pressure low

Ovary
Regulates the menstrual cycle and reproduction

Uterus
Thickens the uterine lining

Bones
Decreases bone breakdown which strengthens bone

Vagina
Causes thickening of the vaginal wall

Testosterone and its functions

Of daily production of testosterone, 25% is produced in the adrenal gland, 25% is produced in the ovaries and 50% is produced from the peripheral conversion of androstenedione, a precursor hormone produced in the ovaries and adrenal gland. Testosterone can also be converted to estrogen. An appropriate balance between testosterone and estrogen is required for successful development of the developing egg. Testosterone receptors have been found in the central nervous system and in bone. Testosterone production in women is one-tenth of that in men. While testosterone has a direct correlation to libido in men, women tend to have more complex factors affecting their sexual motivation.

Chapter 8

Birds & bees revisited
Facts on menstruation

To understand what happens to the body when menstruation stops, it's important to understand how it starts. When a baby girl is born, she has about a million immature eggs stored in tiny, fluid-filled follicles in the ovaries. By the time of puberty, this number drops to 300,000. At puberty, the hypothalamus signals the pituitary gland which turns on the ovaries and starts the process of ovulation, during which one egg is produced every month with regression of many other immature eggs. A woman will release about 400 mature eggs during her reproductive lifetime. The process of ovulation is incredibly complex and requires a virtual orchestra of hormones to produce the symphony called *ovulation*.

Our knowledge of the hormone patterns of the menstrual cycle was first described in 1971 by Dr. Daniel R. Mishell, Jr., a preeminent reproductive obstetrician/gynecologist researcher at the University of Southern California Medical School. The menstrual cycle is divided into two phases: the follicular phase from day one to day 14 and the luteal phase from day 15 to day 28. Day one is the first day of bleeding. On day one, the hypothalamus in the brain sensing that estrogen levels are low, secretes GnRH which signals the pituitary to make FSH to stimulate the growth of follicles. Many immature egg follicles are recruited which produce increasing amounts of estradiol. As day 14 approaches, they all regress except for the "chosen one" which the pituitary has determined is the

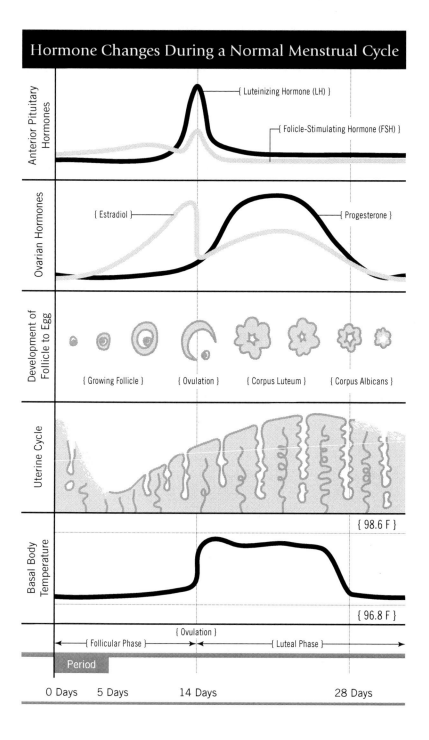

Hormone Changes During a Normal Menstrual Cycle

Anterior Pituitary Hormones
{ Luteinizing Hormone (LH) }
{ Follicle-Stimulating Hormone (FSH) }

Ovarian Hormones
{ Estradiol }
{ Progesterone }

Development of Follicle to Egg
{ Growing Follicle }   { Ovulation }   { Corpus Luteum }   { Corpus Albicans }

Uterine Cycle

Basal Body Temperature
{ 98.6 F }
{ 96.8 F }

{ Ovulation }
{ Follicular Phase }   { Luteal Phase }
Period

0 Days   5 Days   14 Days   28 Days

perfect and best egg. At this point, the hypothalamus signals the pituitary to turn off FSH and to send a hormone messenger in the form of the "LH surge" that signals the ovary to release the chosen egg.

Now the egg must make its journey from the ovary to the open end of the Fallopian tube. Once the egg arrives at one of the Fallopian tubes, it awaits fertilization by a single sperm. Meanwhile, back at the ovary, the luteal phase begins as the empty shell left by the released egg is converted into the corpus luteum that produces large amounts of estrogen and progesterone under the direction of continuing LH. The maximal level of progesterone occurs on day 21 of the menstrual cycle. Progesterone triggers changes in the lining of the uterus, creating a comfortable and safe nest for the egg in case fertilization and conception occurs.

If fertilization occurs, the egg proceeds down to the uterus where pregnancy develops. If fertilization does not occur, after 14 days the egg begins to disintegrate and estrogen and progesterone levels begin to drop. Without the support of these hormones, the lining of the uterus is shed and becomes the menstrual blood that is released each month. So in essence, the menstrual blood represents the cleansing of the uterus which occurs every 28 days. Then the cycle begins all over again and is repeated throughout the woman's childbearing life until the last egg has been released.

Chapter 9

Menstruation begins
The first time for me

Every woman remembers her first menstrual period, the beginning of that awesome passage from girl to young woman.
Some girls can't wait for their period to start, while others feel
afraid or anxious. But for me, it was a shattering experience.
I grew up in a culture where we didn't talk about sexual
things, and I had no idea what was happening to me. I ran
to tell my mother about it. She acted embarrassed and told
me I was now a woman and that's how it would be. She gave
me some pads to wear and that was all the information I was
given.

A friend of mine, Carol, had an even worse experience. She
was worried she'd be bleeding every day for the rest of her life!
A few days later when the bleeding stopped, she was elated,
but then devastated when it came back a month later. Of
course, our friends filled us in on what was going on. I didn't
buy the "being a woman" thing, because it didn't feel very
feminine to have to deal with the cramps and the embarrassing mess, especially when I would bleed through my clothes
and have an "accident" in school. It is no wonder a woman's
menstrual period is often called "the curse."

I remember having very painful menstrual cramps each
month and my doctor trivialized my complaints saying that
was normal. That was before the days of ibuprofen, so I just
suffered through it and went to school. Years later, in my

twenties after I was married, I had an early miscarriage at seven weeks that caused severe uterine cramping. Suddenly, I realized it was the very same sensation as menstrual cramps, only a lot worse. I was furious at the medical establishment for telling me, "it was all in my head." The body doesn't lie. Every sign and symptom means something. It's the language of your body, and it's your body's way of communicating to you that there is a problem.

I now see the menstrual cycle as a fascinating and essential phenomenon that makes each of us a part of the cycle of life. Normal cycles should not be terribly painful and are usually easily managed. If young women in our culture could see it as a celebration, a rite of passage into the family of humanity, I don't think it would be viewed with such disdain.

In fact, early cultures celebrated the first menstruation of young women. The ancient Greeks built temples to house such rituals. African, Asian, and Native American groups honored their young women with elaborate ceremonies. In India, it was a time for rejoicing with gifts, ceremonial baths and feasting. These celebrations and many others were public acknowledgments that the woman was now ready for the responsibilities of marriage and motherhood.

Even though the passage of girl to young woman has been celebrated, until recent years, it has not been understood. For thousands of years, the process of menstruation was cloaked with a tapestry of myth and misinformation. In the 1400s, it was believed sex with a menstruating woman could be fatal. History's first encyclopedia claimed menstrual blood was a deadly poison. It was also believed that if menstruation were to coincide with an eclipse of the moon, incomparable evil would be unleashed. As late as the 19th century physicians were prescribing rather peculiar cures for menstrual cramps. One prescribed a cocktail of sulfuric acid, turpentine, alcohol and brown sugar. Forty drops of the mixture were to be placed in a teacup. After adding water until the teacup was full, the potion was to be consumed immediately. In Victorian times, menstruating women were advised to "wear warm, but loose, clothing, eat plain food, wear good thick-soled shoes and avoid novels which might excite the passions."

Chapter 10

The reproductive years

Problem Periods - It's Not Normal

In the first five to seven years after the first menstrual period and the last ten years before menopause there can be variability in the cycles. Between the ages of 20 and 40 most women's menstrual cycles fall into a familiar pattern of 28-day cycles. A pattern of very short (less than 21 days) or very long (greater than 35 days) time between menstrual periods or skipped periods indicates the woman is not ovulating. Extremely painful or heavy menstrual periods lasting longer than 7 days are also a cause for evaluation.

Sometimes young women with irregular cycles are incorrectly told *"Well, that's just normal for you!"* It is very unfair to trivialize or dismiss these complaints in such patients. Signs and symptoms are your body's way of telling you there's a problem. It's better to find the underlying cause of the menstrual disorder instead of masking it with birth control pills. In many instances birth control pills are prescribed without the woman ever undergoing a diagnostic evaluation. There are consequences to a young woman not having ovulatory cycles. These include bone loss, premenstrual syndrome (PMS), mood disorders, headaches, facial hair, acne, infertility, and a myriad of other symptoms. These symptoms can occur in polycystic ovaries syndrome, hypothyroidism, hyperprolactinemia, all of which are treatable endocrine conditions.

Secondary Amenorrhea - When Your Periods Stop

Secondary amenorrhea is the medical term that is used when a woman who was previously having regular or irregular periods, stops having them. When a woman younger than 40 stops having her periods, it is important to know that this condition is not likely to be menopause. Young women sometimes like the convenience of not having periods and may not seek medical attention. Women with elevations in prolactin and various other coexisting medical problems can have temporary cessation of periods. Women going through severe stress, marked weight loss or extreme exercise may stop having periods. If periods stop for three months or longer, be sure that you undergo a diagnostic evaluation and are not just started on birth control pills or oral contraceptives (OCs) which cause menstrual periods to resume in most women. Such treatment may give women a false sense of security that they are now "normal." Nothing could be further from the truth. OCs in this instance let you know that you have a functioning uterus but nothing about the state of your ovaries. Proper diagnosis and treatment is especially important in younger women concerned about their future fertility.

Birth control pills are a combination of a synthetic estrogen with a synthetic progestin or a synthetic progestin alone. The synthetic estrogen and progestin essentially suppress pituitary LH and FSH that turns off ovulation - the desired effect. The introduction of OCs has transformed women's lives and given us access to effective contraception that facilitates women's ability to integrate careers with family planning. Millions of women tolerate OCs with few side effects. However, women may not always correlate certain side effects with the use of OCs. Women on long-term OCs can have suppression of testosterone resulting in decreased libido and sexual dysfunction.

I recall Andrea, a 25-year-old accountant who came to see me because of sexual dysfunction. She was married to a dental student and they'd had great sex early in their relationship. She started OCs because they didn't want to risk becoming pregnant while her husband was still in dental school. Within six months of starting OCs, she began having very painful intercourse to the point that she would be in tears. She had bleeding every time they had sex. You can imagine what impact this had on her sex drive. Her husband felt horrible and guilty because he didn't want to see his wife in pain. They were both distraught and totally perplexed with the situation. I advised Andrea to stop the OCs, but even after stopping she continued to have vaginal dryness and pain despite having regular periods. After a course of vaginal estrogen, she was finally able to enjoy normal sexual activity.

Oral contraceptives lead to a suppression of testosterone production and an increase in production of sex hormone binding globulin (SHBG) a protein in the blood that binds testosterone leading to lower levels of free testosterone. This occurs more commonly with progestin only contraceptives *(DepoProvera, Norplant,)* and with combined estrogen/progestin OCs containing a strong progestin (e.g. *Ortho 7/7/7, Cyclen, Tricyclen, Yazmin,* and *Yaz.*)

A study in 124 premenopausal women with sexual dysfunction for greater than six months was analyzed by oral contraceptive use. Current birth control pill users had a four times higher level of sex hormone binding globulin (SHBG) compared to women who had never used OCs. Even after stopping OCs for three months, SHBG levels did **not** return to the level of never users. Since elevations in SHBG can lower levels of free testosterone, this was suggested as a possible contributing factor to the sexual dysfunction.

Natural Birth Control - Taking Cues From Your Body

Women today have many choices for contraception but I'm surprised that few know about a more natural, safer form of birth control. This requires that a woman measure her daily temperature to determine the approximate day of ovulation. This method has often been called the "Rhythm Method" and jokes abound about how it doesn't work. The medical term for this technique is the measurement of *basal body temperatures* (BBTs). My belief is that most women who've not had success with this method were never properly instructed. Some physicians unfamiliar with the technique dismiss it as unreliable or believe women are not compliant enough to practice this technique. I have found that people tend to be "down on things they're not up on."

First and foremost, measuring BBTs to practice birth control requires that a woman have regular monthly periods.
If she has irregular periods, it becomes difficult to determine ovulation with any certainty, which makes this method more unreliable. It's also important to use a special basal body thermometer that has units from 96 to 100 degrees, so that changes of one-tenth of a degree can be easily read. This thermometer can be purchased in any pharmacy. *Ovulindex*™ is a good brand and comes with useful forms for charting your temperatures. For detecting these small changes in temperature, I have found mercury thermometers to be more accurate than digital thermometers.

You place the thermometer under your tongue on first awakening before ever getting out of bed or eating or drinking. You chart your daily temperatures this way through the whole month. It's easiest to see the trend if you get up at the same time each day. However, if you have a day when you get up much later you can easily estimate what your temperature would have been at your typical wake-up time by subtracting one-tenth of a degree for each half-hour past your typical wake-up time. For example, if you typically awaken at 6 am and one day sleep in until 10 am, simply subtract 0.8 degree from the 10 am temperature and record the revised temperature. Conversely, if you get up earlier, you use the same ratio but you ADD the additional degrees to estimate what your temperature would have been at the typical wake-up time.

Even though ovulation is exceedingly complex, the concepts for measuring BBTs are simple. The estrogen levels present during the follicular phase before ovulation tend to lower BBTs while the progesterone levels produced in the luteal phase after ovulation tend to raise BBTs. The rise in temperature usually occurs one or two days after ovulation but may vary by three days. Another sign of ovulation is you'll have vaginal discharge of an increased volume of clear, stretchy, slippery mucus. Once the temperature remains elevated for five days, you know ovulation has occurred. Once ovulation has occurred, you know that your period will occur two weeks later.

The benefit of this method of birth control is that you become very familiar with your pattern of ovulation. Essentially once you know when ovulation typically occurs you can abstain or use barrier methods of contraception for four to five days before and after your typical ovulation day. Barrier methods for contraception include spermicides, condoms (male and female), diaphragms and cervical caps. The rest of the month requires no protection and you're not likely to get pregnant. Of course, keep in mind that without protection, you're susceptible to sexually transmitted diseases like herpes. This method is ideal when you're in a stable, long-term relationship with someone you trust.

When you're ready to start your family, you can time sexual activity to one to two days before ovulation to plan the optimal time to get pregnant. You will know you are pregnant when the temperature stays elevated for longer than two weeks after ovulation. You'll see this effect even before traditional pregnancy tests can detect the pregnancy.

A study of 100 fertile couples who conceived without timed intercourse instructions showed a pregnancy rate of 50 percent at three months, 75 percent at six months and 90 percent at one year. Another group of 100 fertile couples who used timed intercourse had a pregnancy rate of 76 percent at one month and 100 percent at seven months. Understanding this concept avoids unnecessary, expensive testing and enables you to plan your pregnancies.

Another benefit of this method is that it gets you in touch with the fascinating rhythm of your body. So many women deny their bodies and forge ahead ignoring subtle symptoms until they become major problems. Our bodies are uniquely equipped to function and recover from illness if we just pay attention to their proper care.

Furthermore, measuring BBTs is very inexpensive, low tech and has no side effects. There are also kits for home use that will detect the LH surge in urine. Recall that LH is luteinizing hormone, the pituitary hormone that triggers the ovary to release the egg. Ovulation kits can be bought in any pharmacy and are somewhat expensive. A useful reliable brand is *Clearblue Easy Read ovulation kit*. You typically start testing your urine one to two days before expected ovulation to plan an optimal time for sexual activity if a pregnancy is desired. However, if you have regular periods, this may not be necessary. If you have been monitoring your basal temperatures for months and you know your ovulation usually occurs on day 14, then begin having sexual activity on days 12 or 13 and you will likely get pregnant.

Let me give you my own personal experience so you can see how effective measuring BBTs can be. As a pharmacist and Assistant Editor for *AHFS-Drug Information*, I was researching the medical literature at the National Library of Medicine in Washington, D.C. for preparation of drug monographs. That was in 1972, long before the Internet, when you had to manually go through voluminous publications like *Index Medicus* that catalogs all the medical journals and literature. I came across an article about determining ovulation with BBTs. I have always been intensely curious about my body so, of course, I delved into that literature.

I successfully utilized this method of birth control for four years before and during my first two years of medical school. In my third year of medical school, I relied on this method to carefully plan a pregnancy. At UCLA, medical students first attend two years of basic science classes followed by two years of rotating clerkships each lasting one to three months. You're given the freedom to plan when and where you want to do your clerkships. I turned in my schedule and planned my delivery due date BEFORE I had even conceived! We were allowed three months off in that two-year interval and so I scheduled three months off to be with my new baby. After breast-feeding and resumption of my periods, I went back to BBTs for contraception until I became menopausal in my forties. For a wonderful book that teaches you more about this method of natural birth control, read *Taking Charge of Your Fertility* by Toni Weschler.

Tubal Ligation - Tying Your Tubes

Women who've already had their children often see tubal ligation as a convenient, risk-free form of birth control. No surgery, however simple, is ever totally free of risks. The euphemistic term "tying your tubes," actually means the tubes are surgically and permanently severed or scarred to prevent the passage of an egg. That is, after all, the goal. Tubal ligation methods may differ in their effectiveness for preventing pregnancy and in the risk of damaging the blood supply to the ovaries.

Many women don't understand that a tubal ligation may cause them to go through perimenopause prematurely. There are structures in the tubes, such as nerves and blood vessels feeding the ovaries, which can be damaged in the procedure. Damage to blood supply can affect the function of the ovaries. At the very least, after tubal ligation, some women begin having heavy bleeding with their periods, and they may also develop symptoms akin to perimenopause. I've seen two women, one in her late twenties and the other in her thirties, who went through menopause after a tubal ligation. While this is exceedingly rare and easily managed, any 28 year old would be psychologically devastated to learn that she is now menopausal.

Should a young woman become perimenopausal after a tubal ligation, it is easily treated, provided the condition is recognized. I have made this diagnosis in women in their thirties who had a tubal ligation months to years prior. They were suffering from a treatable condition but had previously been told, "*Don't be silly. You're too young to be going through perimenopause.*" Overall, tubal ligations are a safe, effective method of sterilization, but it's important to be aware of the risks and to consider the questions with your gynecologist when you're making your decision.

Key Points about Tubal Ligation:

1. Understand this is generally permanent sterilization
2. Study the different types of tubal ligation and discuss with your gynecologist which one is best for you
3. If you develop symptoms of perimenopause after a tubal ligation, have your estradiol and progesterone levels checked on day 21 of your menstrual cycle. FSH, the blood test for menopause, is usually normal

Chapter 11

Perimenopause
The transition into menopause

For most women, menopause doesn't abruptly come out of the blue. There is an interim phase called perimenopause when the body begins its transition into menopause. Lasting anywhere from months to years, it signals that a woman's reproductive years are drawing to a close. At this time, women experience symptoms akin to menopause, although they tend to be milder. These include: hot flashes, mood changes, insomnia, depression, fatigue, acne, memory problems, and sweats.

I've seen several perimenopausal women who develop debilitating headaches with each monthly menstrual cycle. A few of them have suffered monthly migraines since puberty. Physicians call them "menstrual migraines," and they're commonly treated with pain medications, beta blockers or *Imitrex*. They typically occur right before or during the first days of a menstrual cycle. They can also occur mid-cycle, at the time of ovulation. These times in the menstrual cycle are associated with a sharp rise or fall in estradiol which in some women can result in vascular spasm, triggering a migraine. The headaches can usually be prevented by taking a small dose of topical estradiol one day before the anticipated migraine. Topical estradiol can be taken as a cream, gel, spray or patch applied to the skin.

Cathy was a 45-year-old who saw me for perimenopausal symptoms of premenstrual syndrome (PMS), acne and heavy bleeding with her periods. In the course of taking her history, I learned she had suffered severe migraine headaches with her period each month since she was 12 years old. She had been given pain pills, beta blockers and even injectable *Imitrex*, but they never gave her complete relief. Early on in life, she had resigned herself to missing school or work one day each month because of migraines. Imagine her delight when I gave her a single estradiol patch one day before her period, totally eliminating her monthly migraines.

Because the immature egg cells have been present since birth, the mature eggs, which are released in perimenopause, are now forty-something years old. As you might expect, they are not as healthy as the eggs the ovaries released when the woman was 20. Perimenopause is characterized by an uneven rise and fall of estrogen and progesterone that results in significant hormone imbalance. While both hormone levels drop, there's usually more decline in progesterone than estrogen. This imbalance may contribute to the development of heavy menstrual bleeding.

Women in perimenopause often have a normal FSH because they are still producing estrogen and progesterone. Perimenopausal women are often told "everything is normal" when their FSH is normal. A normal FSH simply mean you are not menopausal. It's disconcerting to a woman suffering significant perimenopausal symptoms to be told nothing is wrong. It makes her feel that somehow she is imagining her symptoms. These patients are often prescribed antidepressants or tranquilizers.

An interesting phenomenon occurs, more often in women in their forties but occasionally in older women in their fifties. Beth was a vivacious 54-year-old who had always been a bundle of energy. Her periods had stopped for six months and she presented with classic menopausal symptoms including hot flashes, insomnia, fatigue, and fuzzy thinking. I diagnosed her with menopause because she had an estradiol level of zero and a markedly elevated FSH. I prescribed topical HRT and progesterone and all her symptoms resolved and she was back to her normal self. However, after some months on HRT, she began having breast tenderness, weight gain and fluid retention, symptoms seen with estrogen excess. A repeat blood test showed very high estrogen with a low FSH. Normal doses of replacement HRT will never cause FSH to be low, so I knew she had to be having some spontaneous ovulation. My treatment was to simply stop the HRT and wait until her estradiol level fell again and menopausal symptoms returned. In Beth's case this off/on process continued for several years until finally her last egg was released and she became truly menopausal. When a woman is educated to recognize the symptoms, she knows when to stop or resume HRT.

In perimenopause, menstrual cycle length often lessens from 28 days to 21-25 days. In this phase, the woman may have heavy menstrual bleeding and pass large clots. She may have "flooding" and gush through tampons and several pads. Women typically describe periods where the flow gushes out in one or two days and then abruptly stops a day later. Some women are homebound for one or two days because of concern they will have an "accident" and bleed through their clothes.

Since progesterone levels peak on day 21 of the menstrual cycle, if levels are low at this time, progesterone therapy can be beneficial. Many of the symptoms of PMS and heavy bleeding are caused by the relative imbalance between estrogen and progesterone. When the hormone imbalance is treated early on with progesterone, heavy bleeding is often easily controlled. If progesterone therapy alone is not adequate to control bleeding, oral contraceptives (OCs) may be prescribed through menopause until the periods stop. Women who don't respond to progesterone or OCs should be considered for an endometrial ablation. This is a procedure performed by gynecologists wherein the lining of the uterus, the endometrium, is destroyed. Various types of endometrial ablations, some office-based, are available and should be discussed with the gynecologist. If the bleeding goes on untreated without the benefit of progesterone, OCs or ablation, it can become intolerable and many women develop anemia. At that point, most women are worn down and opt for relieving their symptoms by undergoing a hysterectomy.

Key points to remember about perimenopause:

1. Periods become irregular and tend to become heavier
2. Menstrual cycle length shortens from every 28 days to 21-25 days
3. Women may notice the onset of "PMS" or menopausal symptoms
4. FSH may or may not be normal
5. If FSH is normal, consider checking progesterone on day 21 of the menstrual cycle because it will usually decline before estrogen
6. Progesterone therapy can often alleviate symptoms

Chapter 12

Symptoms of menopause:
Is it hot in here?

The symptoms of menopause are reactions of the body to deficiency of estrogen, progesterone, and/or testosterone. If the change occurs gradually rather than abruptly, the symptoms tend to be milder, because the body has time to adjust and compensate. When symptoms are abrupt, as in surgical menopause, the sudden drop sets off alarms and the woman may experience palpitations, insomnia, nervousness or anxiety. Hot flashes are the typical sign of low estrogen but in many women, hot flashes eventually disappear even without HRT. When low estrogen continues long-term, a woman starts to experience degenerative effects: loss of bone (osteoporosis); brain cells (Alzheimer's); heart disease; dryness of skin, eyes and vagina; as well as many other effects discussed in later chapters. Which tissues are involved and the severity of involvement varies with your genetic susceptibility.

A very few lucky women sail through menopause with minimal symptoms. They have usually been very healthy prior to menopause. However, they are the exception. Most women will have at least some symptoms. See the following list of the signs and symptoms of menopause. These can range from a mild sensation of feeling warm, to a beet red face and drenching sweats that leave the sufferer with wet hair and clothes soaked in sweat. As you can imagine, this can be especially disconcerting to a woman who's in the middle of a business meeting.

A woman may have trouble falling asleep or she may awaken at 3 a.m. unable to get back to sleep. Sometimes she has both! Sleep is the body's time for rejuvenation when new tissues are made or repaired. When this vital restorative time is short-changed, symptoms like chronic fatigue, weight gain, irritability, palpitations, headaches, and migraines can develop.

Dizziness is another symptom that occurs in menopause. Episodes are usually mild and short-lived lasting only a few seconds. Occasionally dizziness may be debilitating. Alice was a 54-year-old woman who came for menopause management. She had been a confident businesswoman and she told me, *"My life is falling apart and I feel like a cripple!"* She was suffering off/on unpredictable bouts of dizziness of such severity that she would have to hold on to the wall to keep from falling. The dizziness had been going on for months, and she'd undergone a very extensive evaluation from a neurologist, a neurosurgeon and a cardiologist. Because all their testing showed NO cause for her dizziness, she was pronounced NORMAL and sent on her way! She had not actually sought me out for the dizziness but rather had resigned herself to her plight. However, after I started her on topical HRT, she never had another bout of dizziness. She was ecstatic to finally be rid of that debilitating symptom! I've never seen another menopausal woman with such severe dizziness but her case taught me to recognize the possibility that it may be related to low estrogen.

Menopausal women often develop body aches and joint pains. In women with rheumatoid arthritis or osteoarthritis, joint pains can be especially troublesome. Muriel was a 48-year-old menopausal woman with the gnarled, disfigured hands seen in some patients with long-term rheumatoid arthritis. She'd had multiple surgeries to restore function to her hands and she prided herself on her independence. She was pain-free and well controlled under the care of her rheumatologist. She worked as an office manager in her rheumatologist's office. At menopause, I had started her on topical estradiol and she felt great with no low estrogen symptoms. Without my knowledge, her rheumatologist urged her to go off hormones because of concerns related to the Women's Health Initiative (WHI). (I'll discuss the WHI later in this book.) She had not come back to see me because she was off hormones.

Six months after stopping HRT, she returned for a second opinion and I was shocked to see the changes in her. She told me, *"Within days of going off the estrogen, I was in agony from a painful flare-up of my arthritis and I had to be hospitalized and treated with high-dose steroids. Even after leaving the hospital, I've been on methotrexate (chemotherapy), but I'm still in pain and can't work."* She had not come back sooner, because she was so fearful of taking estrogen. When I examined her she had open sores on her arms, a common side effect of the methotrexate. She was in constant pain with her arthritis, exhausted from poor sleep and she burst into tears when I came in the room. I felt so badly for her that I gave her a big hug. I told her that HRT is not without risk but reassured her about the differences between Prempro, the drug studied in the WHI, and topical estradiol. She was feeling so poorly she reluctantly agreed to resume her topical estradiol. When her arthritis flare-up resolved within a few days of going on bioidentical HRT, she became a "believer". Shortly thereafter, her rheumatologist was finally able to wean her off the methotrexate. She's never been off her HRT since that time.

This clinical observation has been documented in a two-year study of 88 postmenopausal women with active rheumatoid arthritis randomized to receive calcium and Vitamin D3 either alone or in conjunction with micronized estradiol and progestin. Overall, 65% of the patients in the HRT groups responded to treatment as compared to 40% of the non-hormonal control patients. Treatment with HRT led to better control of inflammation and significant increases in the bone mineral density in the forearm, hip and spine. Furthermore, the women on HRT had slower progression of their arthritis.

A frustrating change that women often see at this time is a tendency to gain weight especially around their waist. For years we've just been told, *"you're just eating too much."* It turns out estrogen in the brain serves as a master switch which controls food intake, energy expenditure and body fat distribution. This lack of estrogen leads to increased abdominal fat, which contributes to insulin resistance. So, there is actually a physiological reason why women start gaining weight in their forties.

One of the most troubling symptoms of menopause is poor memory and decreased focus and concentration. Many women report fuzzy thinking they describe as *"cobwebs in their brain."* Many women who see me are highly educated, successful and very proactive about maintaining their health. Janet was an accomplished CEO and founder of a major company. Her most troubling symptom was her loss of cognitive function, mental clarity and short-term memory. She required an elaborate array of assistants to keep her from forgetting important meetings and facts. She could not leave home without her list of things she had to accomplish that day. Only after she saw the mental symptoms totally resolve with estrogen did she confess to me that she had been secretly terrified she was getting Alzheimer's disease. She was delighted to be back to her old self, excelling in her fast-paced, challenging lifestyle.

Menopausal women off hormones often notice they're more prone to bronchial infections, shortness of breath, and they may even experience a worsening of their singing voice. These symptoms often improve when estrogen is restored. This is explained further in the section on the risks of not taking estrogen.

Menopausal women report feeling sad and depressed for no apparent reason. Women who've never considered themselves "emotional" will suddenly burst into tears over something that would not normally upset them, like watching a TV commercial. They also report mood swings, anxiety and irritability. At the same time, they later feel guilty about jumping on their husbands and children for often trivial reasons. Their families often learn to "stay away from them" at those times and it can cause a great deal of marital discord. I've seen long-term marriages fall apart when neither the husband nor wife understands what's happening. That's why I often encourage their partner to be with them especially at their first patient visit so he can be more supportive.

Women in their forties or fifties are often in the "sandwich" generation with responsibilities for children and husbands while caring for aging parents. It's further compounded if they work outside the home. They may have been previously adept at this type of multitasking but now find themselves "overwhelmed." These are obvious symptoms that get your attention and affect your productivity and well-being.

Mary came in to see me on a myriad of prescription medications. She relayed to me how she'd gotten on all those medicines. In her 40s when her periods started changing, she developed insomnia and depression. She was started on sleeping pills and antidepressants and initially felt better.

When her periods stopped, she was put on Prempro and she gained 30 pounds in the first year. (Recall from my previous discussion above that women without estrogen often gain weight around their middle but it can also be worsened by oral estrogen.) Because of the weight gain and oral estrogen, she was diagnosed with high blood pressure and started on blood pressure medications. From the oral estrogen and weight gain, she developed high cholesterol and had to be started on cholesterol medications. Her weight gain continued and she developed fluid retention often seen with oral estrogen. She was then started on "fluid pills" (diuretics), to deal with her swollen hands and feet. She later developed anxiety and worsening depression at all the changes occurring in her body. Her antidepressants were increased and she was started on strong, anti-anxiety medications (*Xanax*) which made her feel like a zombie throughout the day. She became sluggish throughout the day but she couldn't sleep at night with her sleeping pills and was up doing laundry. Because of her fatigue, she was then started on *Adderal*, which is a potent amphetamine to give her energy! Her weight gain had also caused her to develop reflux and so she'd been given a potent acid blocker, (*Nexium*), which relieved the reflux but gave her bloating and constipation and she was miserable. So in essence she had been put on seven prescription medications when she probably just needed to be treated with topical bioidentical HRT.

I wish I could tell you Mary's story is atypical, but sadly it's an oft-repeated scenario that occurs in all too many women when their symptoms are simply treated with a drug instead of correcting the underlying cause of the symptoms. Often drugs are given to treat the side effects of the initial drugs that were given! In pharmacy circles, this is often called "polypharmacy." After restoring appropriate levels of topical bioidentical estrogen, progesterone and testosterone, many of these prescription medications can often be gradually tapered off.

THE SIGNS AND SYMPTOMS OF PERIMENOPAUSE AND MENOPAUSE

A woman may have all, some or rarely none of the following symptoms:

1. Weight gain, especially around the midriff
2. Sleep disturbances, either falling asleep or staying asleep
3. Hot flashes and/or drenching sweats
4. General heat intolerance
5. Intolerance to extreme heat or cold temperatures
6. "Brain fog" & muddled thinking
7. Poor mental focus & concentration
8. Decreased word retrieval
9. Decreased memory
10. Feeling of being overwhelmed; can't multi-task
11. Depression and feeling blue for no reason
12. Anxiety, irritability and mood swing
13. Decreased interest in sex
14. Vaginal dryness
15. Painful intercourse
16. Change or skipping of periods
17. Periods with heavy bleeding, flooding or clots
18. Crying spells: the "weepies" sometimes for no reason
19. Breast tenderness
20. Fluid retention
21. Fatigue and lack of motivation
22. Headaches or increase in migraine headaches
23. Leakage of urine with sneezing, cough or exercise
24. Constant sense of needing to urinate – urgency
25. Frequent urination day or night

26. Constipation, indigestion and/or bloating
27. Loss of scalp hair
28. Increase in facial hair
29. Acne
30. Joint pains
31. Stiff or aching muscles
32. Dizziness or lightheadedness
33. Irregular heart beat or palpitations
34. Intermittent loss of balance
35. Decreased vision
36. Ringing in the ears
37. Itchy, crawly skin
38. Dry, thinning skin
39. Premature wrinkling
40. Thin, breaking or brittle fingernails

Chapter 13

Natural menopause:
Nature's way

The average age for menopause is 50 to 55. I've seen an occasional woman who has regular monthly periods and then one month has her last period and never has another. However, this is the exception rather than the rule. Typically, women begin with perimenopausal symptoms in their forties. As a woman approaches the end of perimenopause, the periods become lighter and start to become more infrequent. She may skip several months without a period, and then finally the periods stop completely. When the decline in hormones occurs very gradually, a woman may not experience severe symptoms because her body has had time to compensate for the decline in estrogen and progesterone. Often the age of menopause is genetically determined and it is helpful to ask when an older sister or mother went through menopause. A catastrophic, stressful life event can bring on menopause earlier than expected.

Some women are elated when their periods have stopped and experience few adverse symptoms. Other women respond to the loss of estrogen with severe symptoms mentioned in the previous chapter and find it difficult to do their work. Because of such differences, women experiencing great difficulties are sometimes written off as "hysterical" or hypochondriacal, which is very unfair to these women. Overall, there can be tremendous variation in how menopause is experienced by different women. Every time I think I have seen every "variation on the theme," I see yet another woman who is having a slightly different experience.

After menopause, the adrenal glands continue to produce androstenedione, a hormone that is converted in fat cells to another form of estrogen called estrone. This is a reason why obese women may have less severe hot flashes. It also explains why thin women often require higher doses of estrogen to control their low estrogen symptoms.

Chapter 14

Surgical menopause:
Under the knife

Surgical menopause is the removal of both ovaries. A woman undergoing a hysterectomy for benign disease can still maintain her ovaries and this is generally recommended for younger women. In the past, it was customary for women over 40 to be advised to arbitrarily remove their ovaries to "prevent the possibility of ovarian cancer." (This may still be advisable in women with BRCA 1 or 2 mutations, because they are genetically at increased risk for both ovarian and breast cancer.) For the majority of women, removal of both ovaries is no longer recommended, because studies show those who have their ovaries removed have decreased longevity and a seven times higher risk of developing heart disease. Now women are advised to leave the ovaries in unless the woman is over 65 at the time of hysterectomy. Women who choose to have a hysterectomy are elated to be rid of the exhausting heavy bleeding. However, if they choose to also remove the ovaries, they may be opening themselves to a whole new set of post-surgery issues.

Women, especially those under 40, who have their ovaries removed may experience a marked decrease in libido and sexual function. If estrogen therapy does not restore function, adding a small dose of topical testosterone can be beneficial.

In a 2009 study of 29,000 participants in the Nurses' Health Study, 56% of these women who had a hysterectomy for benign disease underwent elective removal of both ovaries. At 24-year follow-up, the incidences of breast and ovarian cancer were lower in these women (30 and 40 fewer cases per 100,000 women, respectively). However, women without ovaries had a higher incidence of heart disease (44 additional cases) and increased deaths from all causes (121 additional deaths per 100,000 women). Women who had ovaries removed before age 50 and did not use HRT, had 176 and 140 additional cases of heart disease and stroke, respectively and 329 excess deaths per 100,000 women.

With surgical menopause, a woman experiences a rapid fall in blood estradiol levels which tends to result in severe hot flashes. Emerging research has linked severe or prolonged hot flashes to an increased cardiovascular risk. A 2010 study reported that women undergoing a rapid transition into menopause have a worsening progression of CIMT than women with natural menopause. Consequently, women undergoing surgical menopause for benign disease should initiate HRT promptly.

I often have women tell me - *"I wish I'd never had my ovaries removed because all my problems started after I had that surgery."* Women with benign disease are sometimes told, *"You've had all your children. You might as well take everything out so you can't get ovarian cancer."*

I recall Gina, a 48-year-old patient who saw me after having undergone a total hysterectomy with removal of the ovaries at age 44. She had been a very accomplished businesswoman. She had enjoyed excellent health all her life and had normal regular periods "like clockwork" each month. She had a great metabolism, ate what she wanted and had always weighed around 110 pounds. In her early forties, she started having heavy bleeding and was diagnosed with fibroids. She sought out an ob-gyn who was an expert in fibroids and a professor at a major medical school far away from Gina's home. The specialist told her she didn't need a hysterectomy and recommended an endometrial ablation at a facility closer to home.

Gina followed up at a facility near her hometown and the physician there insisted she undergo a complete hysterectomy. She was told she needed to remove her ovaries because her mother had breast cancer in her seventies (after many years of Prempro). She reluctantly agreed to the surgery but now states it was the worst decision she ever made. She was started on oral HRT after the surgery but developed a litany of health problems. In the first year after surgery, she gained 50 pounds that led to high cholesterol and high blood pressure. She developed poor sleep, fatigue, and problems with mental focus and concentration. She eventually sold her business because she couldn't function well at work. Her life was totally changed, and she was very remorseful about her decision to remove her ovaries.

I don't want to frighten women who truly need to have their ovaries removed for medical reasons like cancer. It all goes back to carefully considering the benefit-risk ratio. Undergoing a hysterectomy is major surgery and when you have cancer, severe uterine prolapse or any serious condition that has failed medical therapy, it is warranted. However, if you have a benign condition and medical therapy has not been exhausted, please get a second opinion. Do your homework to study all the available options and the potential consequences of each, so you can intelligently discuss your case with your physician.

With surgical removal of the ovaries and uterus, menopause occurs very suddenly. One day a woman is having menstrual cycles and then the day after surgery, she is in menopause. This can be a shock to the system, especially since she must also recover from major surgery. She has to heal and adjust to what has happened both physically and mentally. For some women who have never had children and even those who have, it is a poignant realization that they won't be able to bear children ever again. Other women see it as a loss of their femininity. I think it's important for the patient to know in advance that she is likely to experience these issues after surgery.

Key Points About Surgical Menopause:

1. Most women less than 65 undergoing a hysterectomy for benign disease should not have ovaries removed
2. Most women who've undergone surgical menopause for benign disease should be started on hormone replacement therapy sooner rather than later
3. After surgical removal of the ovaries, once estrogen levels have been restored, most women have improved sexual function if treated with small doses of topical testosterone

Chapter 15

Premature menopause:
When the change comes early

Studies show about eight of every 100 women of childbearing age - about 3.9 million women - go through natural menopause before the age of 40. Sometimes early menopause has a genetic basis and a 2006 study has attributed it to certain genes. In these families premature graying of the hair, sometimes as early as the 20s, is often seen. About 3.2 percent of women with premature ovarian failure also have Addison's disease, an autoimmune disease of the adrenal glands. Addison's disease is easily treated but it can be dangerous for women who don't know they have it. If a genetic basis is suspected these women are well-advised to consider having their families at an earlier age. If your periods stop and you suspect premature menopause, see an endocrinologist to confirm that it is truly menopause and not a temporary cessation from some other abnormality.

Most people are familiar with autoimmune diseases like hypothyroidism and diabetes, in which antibodies destroy the thyroid or pancreas. A similar process can result from antibodies that damage the ovaries. Certain environmental factors may contribute to premature menopause. If a woman has undergone chemotherapy or radiation for cancer, the treatments may permanently damage the ovaries.

The risk of menopause depends on the type and length of treatment (chemotherapy, radiation) and the age of the woman at the time of treatment. The physical symptoms for younger women are much as they would be at age 50, but the emotional impact is often greater. Women with premature menopause often struggle with depression. If they are still childless, they realize their dreams of giving birth are crushed because their reproductive years are over. They often feel somehow "less of a woman." It's like a one-two punch. The body is going through immense changes, and the psyche is being shattered. When menopause comes at such an early age, the woman is subject to a higher risk of heart disease, dementia, osteoporosis and other complications because she is subjected to more years of low estrogen. Because these women will likely receive a longer duration of HRT, it becomes even more important to select topical estrodial, a safer form of HRT.

In an open-label, randomized, controlled crossover trial, women with premature ovarian failure were randomly assigned to either topical estradiol and vaginal progesterone or oral ethinyl estradiol and synthetic progestin. After 28 months, the women receiving topical estradiol and vaginal progesterone had lower blood pressure, better kidney function and less activation of the renin-angiotensin system compared to those receiving oral synthetic estrogens and progestins.

Such findings suggest important implications for the future cardiovascular health of women who undergo premature menopause. The North American Menopause Society and the Endocrine Society recommend that the findings from the Women's Health Initiative (WHI) and the Heart and Estrogen/progestin Replacement Study (HERS) should NOT be applied to women who experience premature menopause.

Key points about premature menopause:

1. Can have a genetic component
2. Can be brought on by chemotherapy, radiation or autoimmune disease
3. Ovarian function may wax and wane especially in the forties
4. Women with menopause prior to age 45 are at increased risk of heart disease, osteoporosis and dementia
5. Because therapy is started at a younger age and for more years, it is advisable to pick the safest therapy: topical estradiol and the addition of cyclic oral or vaginal progesterone if she still has her uterus

To E or not to E...
That is the Questrogen

Chapter 16

The women's health initiative study

It would seem estrogen replacement would be the obvious, reasonable and common sense thing to do. And, in fact, until 2002, hormone therapy centering on estrogen replacement was routinely used to treat menopausal symptoms and protect long-term health.

Then in 2002 something happened that changed everything. A large clinical trial called the **Woman's Health Initiative** (WHI) reported a combination estrogen/progestin (*Prempro*) actually posed more health risks than benefits. These risks were reported to include an increased incidence of heart disease, strokes, pulmonary emboli (blood clots to the lungs) and invasive breast cancer. The benefits included protection against osteoporosis and colon cancer. Soon, because of the ensuing furor, physicians became less likely to prescribe hormone replacement. Up to two-thirds of the women on hormone therapy discontinued its use.

It is critical to know the clinical trial involved the use of a specific product called Prempro, a combination of Premarin and Provera. Premarin is conjugated equine (horse) estrogens and Provera is medroxyprogesterone (MPA). This hormone therapy was selected for the study because it was the most frequently prescribed HRT in the United States.

Now multiple studies have enabled us to understand why
WHI determined there were increased risks with HRT:

1. Age and characteristics of the average participant may have affected the outcome

The average WHI participant had been postmenopausal
without HRT for eight years when she was started on HRT.
Two-thirds of the women were ages 60 to 79 so those participants may have already had heart disease. When they broke
the results down to age and years since menopause, increased
risk of heart disease was seen only in women who started HRT
more than 20 years after menopause.

A 2007 re-analysis of the WHI data by age and years since
menopause showed that women who started either Premarin
or Prempro within 10 years of menopause had no statistically
significant increase or decrease in risk of heart disease. (This
essentially translates to no benefit in protection against heart
disease.) Among women ages 50 to 59, a similar non-signifi-
cant trend was observed for improvement in total mortality
but the risk of stroke was elevated regardless of years since
menopause. Other limitations that may affect generalizing
these findings to newly menopausal women is that 34% of
WHI participants were obese, 50% were current or past smokers and women with low estrogen symptoms were excluded
from the study. So WHI was not designed to assess the impact
of HRT on menopausal symptoms which is the reason most
women are given HRT.

2. Continuous combined estrogen/progestin (Prempro) was used in WHI.

In addition to the increased risk of heart disease, breast cancer, strokes and pulmonary emboli, more recent reanalysis of

the data has also shown increased risks of dementia, incontinence, and gallstones. The addition of a daily progestin seems to confer these increased risks. This issue will be further explained in the section that addresses the risks of estrogen.

3. Oral hormones were used

WHI patients with a hysterectomy on oral Premarin alone were reported to have an increased incidence of strokes, pulmonary emboli and gallstones after 7.1 years. Premarin did not increase heart disease but offered no protective effect on heart disease or colon cancer as compared to placebo.

A 2006 study of the WHI group on Premarin showed no increased risk of invasive breast cancer after 7.1 years. There was actually a trend toward a lower incidence of breast cancer that was totally unexpected. (See Chapter 19 for more discussion on this association) However, a re-analysis of the WHI data in 2008 showed that the Premarin group had a more than two-fold increase in the risk of benign proliferative breast disease. Since proliferative breast disease is associated with an increased risk of breast cancer, the authors concluded, "Longer follow-up of the trial participants may help to resolve the apparent contradiction between this finding and the lack of increased breast cancer seen in the initial study. Premarin had no protective effect against memory loss or dementia. Some of these adverse effects appear related to the effect of oral hormones on the liver. This issue will be further explained in the section addressing the risks of estrogen.

When WHI was published, I saw the results as justification for why I've always used topical rather than oral hormones. The adverse effects seen in WHI gave further proof of the consequences of defying the basic physiology of the body. Why give a synthetic estrogen and progestin when you can easily give the very same hormones intrinsic to your body? Why vary the body's natural cycle of two weeks of progesterone each month by giving progesterone daily?

It's been known since the 1970s that oral estrogen causes a myriad of side effects because the liver has to process the excess estrogen before it is delivered to the rest of the body. Topical estradiol therapy was first introduced in the US in 1986 to avoid these adverse effects. I was glad to see a study that validated my continuing use of topical estradiol. However, I was dismayed when WHI was used as a justification to condemn all hormone replacement therapies. Once I carefully explained the difference between Prempro and topical estradiol to my patients, very few asked to go off their hormones.

In the following chapters entitled, *Increased Risks From Oral Estrogens* and *Increased Risks of Continuous Combined Oral Estrogen/Progestin*, I will describe in greater detail the reason why Premarin and Prempro cause increased risks. I've summarized these risks in the key points that follow this WHI chapter.

Key points about the Women's Health Initiative

1. Women who were 20 years past menopause may already have had heart disease, and adding Prempro made it worse
2. Participants included increased numbers of obese smokers
3. Oral hormones (Premarin, Prempro) cause increases in blood clots, strokes, and gallstones through the "first-pass" effect on the liver
4. Adding daily Provera to the Premarin neutralizes many of the benefits of estrogen
5. Premarin and Prempro increase the risk of heart disease, blood clots, and breast cancer when initiated in woman 10 years past menopause

6. Premarin and Prempro increases the risks of pulmonary emboli
7. WHI results should be attributed only to the specific formulations of oral Premarin and Prempro and should not be extrapolated to all HRT newly menopausal women
8. Premarin and Prempro can cause weight gain, sexual dysfunction, gall bladder disease and stones, insulin resistance, metabolic syndrome, and migraine headaches
9. Prempro can worsen dementia, cognitive function, urinary incontinence, and hearing loss

Chapter 17

The timing hypothesis and
the case for natural hormones

❁

It has been suggested that to protect the heart, hormone therapy needs to be started within 10 years of menopause and continued for 10 or more years. This has been termed *"the timing hypothesis."* The thinking was that hormone therapy might be beneficial when started soon after menopause and harmful when started many years after menopause because blood vessel damage had already occurred. When the WHI investigators proposed this hypothesis, they suggested that "health care providers need not be unduly concerned about coronary risk" when HRT was given for short-term relief of menopausal symptoms.

However in a 2009 study, WHI researchers published new data from both the WHI randomized trial of 17,000 women and from an ongoing WHI observational study of 100,000 women that included those who had started HRT soon after menopause.

Their findings showed that both estrogen alone (Premarin) and estrogen/medroxyprogesterone (Prempro) adversely affected risk of heart disease, stroke and blood clots, regardless of whether HRT was started less than five years or greater than five years after menopause. Women who initiated either HRT less than five years after menopause had a substantially higher risk for invasive breast cancer than those who initiated HRT after five years.

A 2009 French E3N cohort study of 53,310 postmenopausal women reported that women who initiated estrogen/progestin HRT within three years of menopause, and took HRT for two years, had a 54% higher risk of breast cancer compared to those who never took HRT. Of note, however, they reported that this increased risk of breast cancer was not seen in women given estradiol/progesterone within three years of menopause.

A 2010 study published by lead author, Dr. Sengwee Toh from Harvard analyzed only the data for heart disease and found that Prempro slightly increased the risk of heart disease in women who initiated therapy within the first two years after menopause but the increase was not statistically significant and disappeared after six years of use. Dr. Toh suggested these effects might be unique to the particular hormones used in WHI.

Oral synthetic estrogen and oral estrogen/synthetic progestins likely have different effects than estradiol and progesterone. Despite the above findings, there may be still justification for the timing hypothesis. Primate studies, which predominantly utilize estradiol therapy, have shown a 70% reduction in atherosclerosis when estradiol is started shortly after menopause. We have previously mentioned the myriad beneficial effects of estradiol on cells throughout the body. Estradiol has beneficial effects on blood vessels in the heart, kidney, and brain which include dilating blood vessels, inhibiting the development of plaque, antioxidant effects which prevents LDL deposits, and increasing beneficial HDL while decreasing LDL production.

Are we to believe that estradiol and progesterone normally produced by a woman during her reproductive years that provide beneficial, wide-ranging protective actions, suddenly become a risk when we give them therapeutically at menopause? A more likely explanation is differences in effectiveness between estradiol and the synthetic horse estrogens found in Premarin and Prempro. The following studies support this reasoning.

A heart benefit of estradiol occurs by increasing production of nitric oxide, a substance that dilates blood vessels. A 2010 study comparing the effects of horse estrogen (*Premarin*) and estradiol in human blood vessel cells showed that horse estrogen was much less effective at increasing nitric oxide production than estradiol. At menopause, loss of estradiol leads to an increase in blood pressure that contributes to postmenopausal hypertension. Numerous studies show that topical estradiol, but not oral horse estrogen, is associated with reductions in blood pressure.

A positron emission tomography (PET) scan is a diagnostic imaging scan that uses low-dose radioactive sugar to measure functional brain activity. PET scans can be used to demonstrate patterns associated with Alzheimer's disease. In a 2010 study, 53 postmenopausal women at increased risk for Alzheimer's disease and previously on estrogen at least a year underwent a baseline PET scan. Women taking estradiol performed three standard deviations higher in verbal memory than women taking Premarin. Women taking an estrogen/ progestin combination pill (Prempro) had lower brain metabolism than women taking estrogen alone.

The actions of estradiol and progesterone, like all hormones, involve intricate physiological complexity. Furthermore, accumulating data shows convincing evidence that many of the beneficial actions of estradiol result from its conversion to downstream *byproducts* of estradiol that act on the cardiovascular and renal systems, independent of estrogen receptors.

These estradiol byproducts, specifically catecholestradiols and methoxyestradiols, protect the heart, blood vessels, and kidneys from disease. Since horse estrogen contains very little estradiol, it cannot be converted to these beneficial downstream byproducts

In addition to protecting blood vessels in the heart and kidneys, 2-methoxyestradiol also inhibits growth of multiple cancer cells including ER-positive and ER-negative breast cancer cells, inhibits angiogenesis (growth of new vessels which feed cancer) and prevents tumor growth. Clinical trials are under way studying the use of 2-methoxyestradiol as an anti-cancer drug.

Determining the presence of these beneficial byproducts is another reason to evaluate estradiol metabolism that we will discuss in a later chapter. If your own body has the ability to produce such a beneficial byproduct, wouldn't you want to know if your liver is making adequate amounts? I tell my patients to think of 2-methoxyestradiol as a "twofer" because that one byproduct gives you two protective benefits against both heart disease and cancer. Every woman who loves shopping appreciates that concept!

An important study called the Kronos Early Estrogen Prevention Study (KEEPS), was started in 2005 and will conclude in 2012. KEEPS is comparing two groups of women on oral estrogen (Premarin) or topical estradiol who are also taking cyclic progesterone. Women included in the study have to be within three years of menopause. They will be monitoring the rate of change of *carotid intima-media thickness* (CIMT) an ultrasound test that monitors for improvement or progression of heart disease. CIMT is discussed more extensively in the section on heart disease in Chapter 22.

WHI is an important study that showed Premarin and Prempro carry a higher risk of adverse effects and are not the safest choices for HRT. However, the adverse effects seen in WHI should be attributed only to the formulation and regimens used in that study. They should not be extrapolated to include all other types of HRT. Since Premarin and Prempro (oral horse estrogen) contain very little estradiol, they cannot be converted in the liver to the beneficial byproducts mentioned above. This may explain why Premarin and Prempro instead produce unwanted adverse effects. It goes back to respecting the basic physiology of the body whenever possible. Why give a synthetic substitute when we can easily restore the deficient hormone that is intrinsic to the body?

Scientific organizations like the North American Menopause Society, the American Association of Clinical Endocrinologists and the Endocrine Society have to wait to make definitive recommendations until extensive large *randomized clinical trials* (RCTs) show clear benefits and risks from any one HRT regimen. RCTs are given more importance than observational studies in dictating published standards. However, from my perspective, if large observational studies suggest a particular HRT regimen may be safer, I feel compelled to act on that information, especially when it supports my clinical observations.

Chapter 18

A woman's decision to take HRT is greatly affected by whether she is having bothersome symptoms. Understandably, if a woman is experiencing minimal symptoms, she may be less inclined to take estrogen. Women with a family history of cancer, heart disease, Alzheimer's disease, or osteoporosis should carefully weigh each of these factors with her physician.

There is much you can do yourself to improve your health and lessen risks. Many chronic diseases are made worse by poor life-style choices. Eating nourishing foods, exercising on a regular basis, getting adequate sleep, maintaining a healthy weight, not smoking and having little or no alcohol are all healthy habits that greatly fortify the ability of your body to stay healthy.

We all know these benefits but their importance often gets diluted by the latest new drug that promises results by just taking a pill. I challenge myself and my patients by reminding them that each of these beneficial activities, especially exercise, is like medicine with far-ranging benefits on your metabolism. A study of 23,153 participants ages 35 to 65, followed for 7.8 years, studied the effect of four factors: never smoking, being non-obese, performing 3.5 hours or more of exercise per week and eating a nutritious diet. Participants who adhered to all four factors at the beginning of the study had a 78% lower risk of developing a disease like diabetes, myocardial infarction (heart attack), stroke or cancer as compared to participants who did not follow these factors.

If we strive to follow these lifestyle habits, we enhance therapies that physicians can offer. Some individuals are blessed
with good genetics but no matter how good your genes are,
if you don't follow a healthy lifestyle, eventually the system
breaks down. Become informed, proactive, and accountable
for your actions and omissions. A knowledgeable, engaged
patient working with her physician increases the likelihood of
achieving her health goals.

Statistics

For the average woman, it can be confusing to assess statistical terms like statistical significance, lifetime risk and relative
risk. Understanding these terms will make it easier for you to
evaluate clinical studies.

Statistical significance

This refers to the likelihood that a particular event occurred
solely from chance or coincidence. The likelihood of a particular event is given a probability value (p-value) and a level
of 0.05 or less is considered statistically significant. When a
study's results shows a p-value of 0.05, it means that there
is a 5% chance that the study's results are due to chance or
coincidence and a 95% chance that it occurred as a result of
the therapy that was being studied. The lower the p-value the
more likelihood that the therapy given produced the results.

Lifetime risk

This represents the probability of developing a particular
disease over the course of your entire life. For example, a
woman's lifetime risk of developing ovarian cancer is 1.7%.

This means that in a group of 100 women followed from birth to age 85, fewer than two women will get ovarian cancer. Another way of expressing lifetime risk: at age 85 a woman has a 1 in 59 risk of developing ovarian cancer and a 58 in 59 risk of *not* developing that cancer.

Absolute Risk

This is a term that compares the incidence of a risk in different groups and it is straightforward to understand. For example, the annual risk of developing gallstones is 47 cases out of 10,000 women who never take HRT. In women who take oral estrogen, the risk of gallstones increases to 78 cases in 10,000 women. While this is a significant increase, there are still 9922 women who don't get gallstones from oral estrogen. It is easier to evaluate risks if you can compare the absolute differences between women who take HRT and those who do not. For example, if one person in 1000 in one group and two persons of 1000 in another group gets the result, the absolute risk is tiny but the second group has a 50% increased risk. Whenever possible, I have presented the data in absolute terms to provide a context for the differences.

Relative Risk

The term, *"relative risk"* (RR) is commonly used in studies to compare the risk in two different groups. For example, we can apply the above two figures for absolute risk of gallstones with and without oral HRT and describe them in terms of relative risk. The group that never takes HRT is given a RR value of 1.00 that represents the 47 cases that naturally occur. The group who takes HRT has 78 cases of gallstones. This group is assigned a RR of 1.66. This value is derived by dividing 78 cases with the therapy by 47 cases without the therapy.

RR simply compares the difference in risks between the group that received HRT and one that did not. A well-meaning reporter might give a sound bite like oral HRT increases your risk of gallstones by 66%. This is a true statement but a woman not familiar with statistics might think that 66 women out of 100 who take oral estrogen will get gallstones! RR simply means that the small baseline RISK (47 cases in 10,000) increases by 66% with HRT (78 cases in 10,000) but gallstones are still not a frequent occurrence.

If a RR is greater than 1.00, it suggests that giving a particular drug increases the risk while a RR less than 1.00 decreases the risk of a particular drug. If the RR is equal to 1.00, than there is no benefit or risk to the group receiving the drug.

A Call for Fair and Balanced Risk Assessment

Risk assessment is sometimes better understood by applying it to common activities we all experience. For example, a events risk of 1 in 10,000 is about equal to the chance of dying from taking 100 flights on regularly scheduled jet airliners. Most of us accept this degree of risk because we desire the benefit gained from making that plane trip. This same concept applies when considering adverse drug reactions.

The benefit-risk ratio must always be considered when selecting any drug. No therapy, especially a prescription medication, ever has 100% benefits with zero risks. Adverse risks are easier to grasp in terms of absolute risks to a given group. Physicians are more likely to prescribe a drug when it provides multiple benefits and serious risks are rare or very rare.

The World Health Organization Council provides a gauge to evaluate the significance of adverse drug reactions (ADR.)

"VERY COMMON" if ADR occur in 1 or more of 10 people taking the drug;

"COMMON" if ADR occur in 1 or more of 100 people but less than 1 in 10.

"UNCOMMON" if ADR occur in 1 or more of 1000 people but less than 1 in 100

"RARE" if ADR occur in 1 or more of 10,000 people but less than 1 in 1000

"VERY RARE" if ADR occur in less than 1 of 10,000 people.

In a compelling 2008 review of multiple studies, Dr. Howard N. Hodis, a cardiologist in the preventive cardiology unit at USC School of Medicine, compared the risks and benefits of hormone replacement therapy for preventing heart disease with that of drugs like "statins," cholesterol-lowering drugs, commonly used for heart disease.

A meta analysis of 30 randomized controlled trials comparing women taking HRT to those on no HRT showed a 40% reduced mortality in women who started HRT younger than 60 or within 10 years of menopause. Contrast this to cholesterol-lowering drugs, like statins, which have not been shown to reduce mortality in women.

Most women and physicians are fearful of the increased risk of breast cancer from estrogen but few are aware that statins have a similar risk of breast cancer. Physicians routinely prescribe statins that increase breast cancer risk despite the fact that it has not been shown to reduce mortality in women. Dr. Hodis points out that these risks from statins and other commonly used drugs are considered "acceptable." Yet these same risks from HRT have been given inordinately greater negative exposure. This type of focus even prompted the FDA to issue a "black box" warning for estrogen, whereas no such such requirement exists with other drugs with a similar risk.

The point is not to advocate or criticize the use of one drug or another but to use some common sense and put the risks and benefits in clinical perspective. The risks of breast cancer from statins or HRT are RARE and should be considered in light of potential benefits. These are important considerations for both the patient and her physician so they can make decisions that are right for her as an individual.

Perception Versus Reality

Another important consideration of risk assessment comes from women themselves. By far, women's greatest fear of HRT is the possible increase in the risk of breast cancer. Yet the actual risks of other diseases resulting from NOT taking HRT are actually far greater.

The following graph compares deaths from heart disease to deaths from strokes, lung cancer, chronic lower respiratory disease, Alzheimer's and breast cancer.

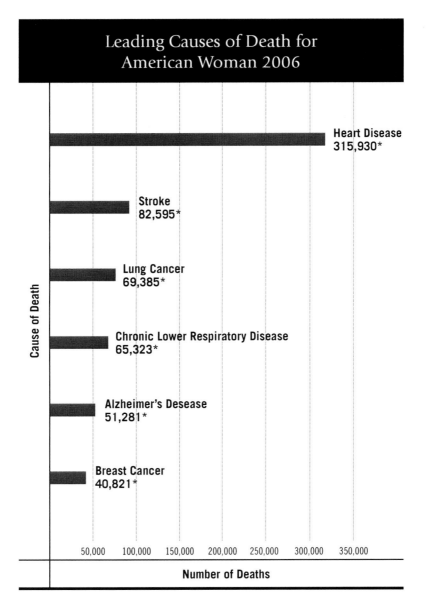

Leading Causes of Death for American Woman 2006

Heart Disease
315,930*

Stroke
82,595*

Lung Cancer
69,385*

Chronic Lower Respiratory Disease
65,323*

Alzheimer's Desease
51,281*

Breast Cancer
40,821*

Cause of Death

50,000 100,000 150,000 200,000 250,000 300,000 350,000

Number of Deaths

One in four women dies from heart disease. It's the #1 killer of women, regardless of race or ethnicity. It also strikes at younger ages than most people think and the risk rises in middle age. Two-thirds of women who have heart attacks never fully recover.

*As reported by CDC (2006), National Vital Statistics Reports 57(14): pp 1-135, April 17, 2009

In a survey of 1000 women ages 45 to 64, 61% said the disease they feared most was cancer, primarily breast cancer. Only 9% said they feared heart disease, the disease most likely to kill them. **Heart disease kills more women each year than the next 16 causes of death combined, including diabetes, all forms of cancer, AIDS and accidents. Because women tend to over-estimate the risk of breast cancer it's important to put this risk in proper perspective.**

Considering Breast Cancer Risk Factors

With regard to breast cancer risks, there are factors that are not within your control and those which are modifiable. The latter are the areas where you can have the most impact.

Risk Factors (Mostly) Not Under Your Control

Besides being female, the most important risk factor for breast cancer is increasing age. This is understandable because as your immune system ages, it becomes less effective at protecting you against cancer. The widely touted figure of one in eight women having a "lifetime" risk of developing breast cancer does not apply until a woman reaches the age of 85. On the other hand, the chance of never having breast cancer by 85 is seven in eight.

The following graph was developed by the *National Cancer Institute* and shows a woman's risk of developing breast cancer at different ages.

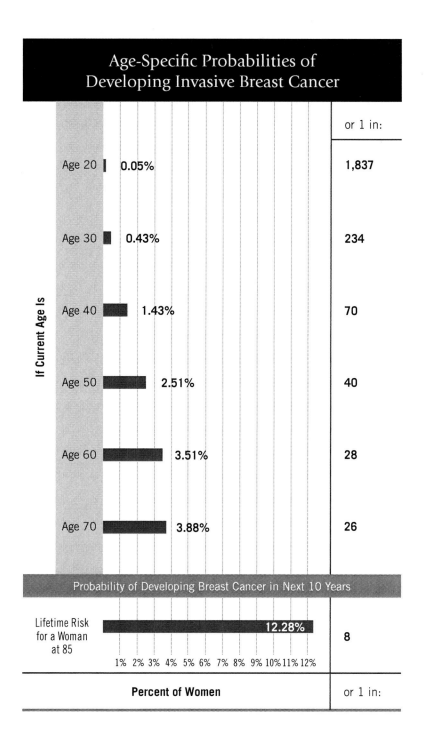

The life-long cumulative exposure of the breasts to estrogen caused by early onset of periods and later menopause is a factor that increases the risk of breast cancer. Having a first pregnancy by age 25 confers a protective effect on the breast and lowers a woman's risk of breast cancer by 10 percent. However, the general trend is for American women to marry later, and early pregnancy is often not an option. A 2007 study found the relative risk of developing breast cancer in post-menopausal women with dense breasts was 400% higher than in women with fatty, non-dense breast tissue. It used to be thought that the risk of dense breasts was simply a reflection of higher levels of circulating estrogen. However, this study showed that women with dense breasts who also had higher levels of circulating estrogen or testosterone had a 200% further increase in risk of breast cancer suggesting these are two independent factors.

A positive family history of breast cancer is seen in only 15 to 20% of women with breast cancer. The risk is increased if there are multiple first-degree female relatives with breast cancer or if the relative's cancer occurred before age 40. BRCA are breast cancer genes which pose no risk to a woman when they function normally. If however, the genes transform to BRCA-1 or -2 mutations, cancer risk increases. Although less than 10% of all breast cancers are linked to these genetic mutations, women with these mutations are at very high risk for breast cancer.

According to 2005 guidelines issued by the *US Preventive Services Task Force*, the following family history patterns are associated with an increased risk of BRCA-1 or -2 mutations: For non-Ashkenazi Jewish women, these patterns include 2 first-degree relatives with breast cancer, 1 of whom received the diagnosis at age 50 years or younger; a combination of 3 or more first- or second-degree relatives with breast cancer regardless of age at diagnosis; a combination of both breast and ovarian cancer among first- and second-degree relatives; a first-degree relative with bilateral breast cancer; a combination of 2 or more first- or second-degree relatives with ovarian cancer regardless of age at diagnosis; a first- or second-degree relative with both breast and ovarian cancer at any age; and a history of breast cancer in a male relative. For women of Ashkenazi Jewish heritage, an increased-risk family history includes any first-degree relative (or 2 second-degree relatives on the same side of the family) with breast or ovarian cancer.

A blood test to detect BRCA genetic mutations is available but the *US Preventive Services Task Force* recommends referral for genetic counseling before BRCA testing.

Women with positive BRCA genetic mutations are advised to have clinical breast exams every six months and yearly mammograms. Surveillance for ovarian cancer includes yearly transvaginal ultrasounds and measuring cancer antigen (CA)-125 blood levels.

Preventive mastectomy (removal of healthy breast tissue) - reduces breast cancer risk by 90% and removal of ovaries reduces ovarian cancer risk by 90%.

While these risks are generally not modifiable, knowing them may enter into your decision about whether to take HRT. It also will make you more diligent about addressing the factors that you can change and monitoring for early detection.

RISK FACTORS YOU CAN MODIFY
TO DECREASE YOUR RISK

Obesity

Obesity and weight gain during adult life increases risk of postmenopausal (but not premenopausal) breast cancer because fat tissue increases estrogen levels. The adverse effect of obesity on breast cancer is strongest in women who do not use HRT. In the Nurses' Health study, women gaining 22 pounds or more after menopause increased their risk by 18% while losing at least 22 pounds lowered their breast cancer risk by 57%.

Alcohol Intake

A meta-analysis of over 40 epidemiologic studies showed that drinking 2 drinks a day may increase the risk of breast cancer by 21%. The Million Women study published in 2009 showed than drinking even 1 drink a day increases the risk of breast cancer. Each additional alcoholic drink regularly consumed per day was associated with 11 additional breast cancers per 1000 women. Even though alcohol has been previously associated with cardiac benefits, Michael Lauer MD of the US National Heart, Lung and Blood Institute editorialized that the excess cancer risk seen in this study may outweigh the benefits.

Exercise

Several studies show that exercising 45 to 60 minutes daily for 5 or more days per week reduces the risk of breast cancer in postmenopausal women. One study showed regular physical activity, regardless of intensity, may reduce the risk of breast cancer in postmenopausal women.

Breast Feeding

Breast feeding has consistently been shown to lower the risk of breast cancer. A study of 47 epidemiological studies in 50,302 women with breast cancer and 96,973 women without breast cancer showed that the incidence of breast cancer was reduced by 4.3% for every 12 months of breast feeding. The protective effect is thought to be related to the delay in resumption of ovulatory cycles from breast-feeding.

Fibrocystic Breast Disease

Women diagnosed with fibrocystic breast disease (FBD) and a family history of breast cancer are at increased risk for breast cancer if a breast biopsy shows certain proliferative changes even though the pathology was benign for cancer. Symptoms of FBD may sometimes be improved with therapies including evening primrose oil, vitamin E, iodine, and diindolemethane, and avoiding caffeine.

Vitamin D Deficiency

Two 2010 meta-analysis studies showed that maintaining sufficient levels of serum vitamin D protects against breast cancer. One study showed a 41% reduction in breast cancer risk in case-control studies. The other study showed among those with the highest intake of vitamin D, the risk of breast cancer was reduced by 45% compared to those with the lowest intake of vitamin D.

Laboratory studies also support this protective action against breast cancer through several mechanisms. A 2010 review article reported that a vitamin D byproduct promotes *apoptosis* (programmed self-destruction) of breast cancer cells, decreases excess estrogen production and has anti-inflammatory actions.

Vitamin D is the "sunshine vitamin" and you can often get adequate levels of vitamin D by regularly receiving mid-day sun exposure in the late spring, summer, and early fall, exposing as much of the skin as possible for 20-30 minutes but being careful not to burn. Individuals with dark skin may need up to six times longer exposure time because of less absorption. In winter, it's often more challenging to get adequate levels from sun exposure alone.

For those who cannot get adequate sun exposure, vitamin D supplementation is recommended. The *Canadian Cancer Society* recommends a minimum of **1000 IU of vitamin D3** but much higher levels are often needed. Dr. John Cannell, Director of the Vitamin D Council suggests adults often need around **5000 IU of vitamin D3**. He suggests monitoring blood 25-hydroxy Vitamin D to ensure adequate levels. Dr. Cannell also emphasizes the importance of other nutrients such as magnesium, zinc, vitamin K2, boron and a small amount of vitamin A, which improve the utilization of vitamin D.

Abnormal estrogen metabolism

This section may seem a little technical but do not gloss over it because it's it is important for you to understand. Or at least come back to review it later. Anything taken into your body such as medicines or hormones produced by the body, has to be processed by the liver which is responsible for their orderly disposition. The liver is an important organ that has to break down any hormone, food, medicine or chemical you take into your body. Toxic materials are broken down into byproducts that can be easily removed from the body. The breakdown of these substances sometimes produces substances more beneficial to the body. For example, whether you're still making estradiol or taking it, effects of estradiol occur from the estradiol itself and other effects occur through chemical reactions in the liver that produce byproducts from the processing of estradiol. The medical term for these byproducts is "downstream metabolites."

Estradiol is broken down in the liver to various byproducts called 4-hydroxyestrone (4-byproducts) and 16-hydroxyestrone (16-byproducts.) Excess levels are associated with a higher risk of breast cancer, ovarian cancer, and uterine cancer so we call these the "bad" estrogens. Estradiol is also converted to 2-hydroxyestrones (2-byproducts) that carry a lower risk of cancer and these are called the "good" estrogens. A small amount of the 16-byproducts is necessary to maintain strong bones. The goal is a healthy balance between these three estrogen byproducts. The 4-byproducts are the most harmful so the liver has a chemical process called methylation to neutralize these bad estrogens.

In 2006, a review article in the *New England Journal of Medicine* gave an extensive review of the literature supporting the role of estrogen metabolites as cancer initiators. While this may not be the only cause of these cancers, it is a risk factor that can often be modified with healthy lifestyle and supplements. There are not yet extensive randomized controlled trials showing benefit from these therapies. However, if the therapy is low-risk and possibly beneficial, why would we NOT want to consider this therapy to reduce cancer-promoting byproducts to improve the safety of estrogen therapy?

The relative amounts of "bad" estrogens can be improved with lifestyle intervention such as exercise, flaxseed, improved nutrition and the intake of cruciferous vegetables. Cruciferous vegetables include broccoli, cauliflower, cabbage, kale, and brussel sprouts. For women who may not consume adequate amounts of these vegetables, nonprescription supplements called *diindolemethane* (DIM) and indole-3-carbinol (I3C) contain the active protective ingredients of these vegetables.

In addition, recent studies in the cardiology literature show that when the 2-byproduct undergoes methylation, it is converted to 2-methoxyestradiol which protects against heart disease and has an anti-cancer effect. (Studies in the oncology literature are underway to study the potential use of this byproduct as an anti-cancer drug) When deficient, this beneficial byproduct can often be increased by use of supplements. Why would we NOT want to increase production of this beneficial byproduct to maximize the full benefit of estradiol therapy?

Methylation can be improved with nonprescription supplements including vitamin B12, folic acid, zinc, resveratrol, N-acetylcysteine, trimethylglycine, and S-adenosyl-methionine (SAM-e). I would advise against any of the dietary supplements unless you are working with a knowledgeable professional who can monitor your levels and advise you on appropriate doses of these products. The estradiol byproducts can be measured in the urine. The test requires collecting the first morning urine made over the previous 8 hours, sending a sample of urine from that total volume and indicating the total volume. After therapy to improve estrogen metabolism has been initiated, follow-up testing is repeated in three months to assess whether there has been improvement. Thereafter testing is done on a yearly basis. With correction of estrogen metabolism, women often report reduction in breast tenderness, PMS and other menstrual related complaints. It also gives us another parameter to monitor to improve safety and enhance the full benefit of estradiol.

SCREENING FOR BREAST CANCER -
THE IMPORTANCE OF EARLY DETECTION

Tumor size greatly affects mortality. The smaller the tumor, the more likely it is to be confined to the breast and therefore more responsive to treatment. In a study of 83,686 cases of women with primary breast cancer with tumor sizes ranging from 0.3 cm to 5 cm, and no lymph node involvement, the smallest tumors were associated with a mortality of 10% while the larger tumors were associated with a mortality of 25%. In women with tumor sizes ranging from 0.3 cm to 5 cm and positive lymph nodes, those with the smallest tumors had a 20% mortality and those with the larger tumors had a 40% mortality. Studies show improved mortality when breast cancer is detected as a small lesion, especially if it's less than 2 cm.

Mammography

In November 2009, the *US Preventive Services Task Force* (USPSTF) issued new guidelines for screening mammograms for women with no signs or symptoms of breast cancer. They recommend screening every two years in women ages 50 to 74. In women 75 years or older insufficient evidence exists to recommend routine screening. USPSTF recommends against routine screening of women aged 40 to 49 years because the risks of mammograms outweigh the benefits. These recommendations do not apply to women 40 years or older who are at increased risk or breast cancer by virtue of a known underlying genetic mutation or a history of chest radiation. USPTSF recommends against routine clinical breast examination (CBE) unless the physician is committed to performing a more structured, standardized examination.

Various organizations are not in agreement with the USPSTF recommendations to not screen women ages 40 to 49. This contention has been further strengthened by a 2010 breast cancer screening study of 600,000 Swedish women that found annual mammography screening of women in their 40s reduces breast cancer death rate in these women by nearly 30%.

The American Cancer Society (ACS) in 2003 recommended annual mammography and clinical breast examination beginning at age 40. In 2003, *The American College of Obstetrics and Gynecology* (ACOG) recommended mammography every 1 to 2 years for women 40 to 49 and annually after the age of 50. ACOG recommends CBE and breast self-examination (BSE) for all women.

Breast tissue in younger women less than 40 tends to be both firmer and denser, making it more opaque to X-rays so that tumors are less likely to be detected. High risk women, especially those with BRCA1 or BRCA2 gene mutations or with a family history of breast cancer are advised against undergoing mammograms before the age of 20. Research presented in 2009 showed that women who underwent five or more annual mammograms starting at age 20, had a 2.5 times higher risk of breast cancer than those women not exposed to the mammography radiation.

It's also important to emphasize that mammography can sometimes fail to detect tumors which can be felt on physical exam by the patient or the physician especially in women with dense breasts. Other imaging techniques include magnetic resonance imaging (MRI), ultrasound, and thermography. However, mammography remains the standard procedure for detecting breast cancer.

Breast Examination

Physicians perform the *clinical breast examination* (CBE) as part of the routine physical and ACOG and ACS recommend yearly examinations for women age 40 and older. Periodic breast exams every three years are advised in women ages 20 to 40 especially if they have firm/dense breasts or a strong family history of breast cancer. While not an official recommendation, ACS suggests that women begin practicing *breast self-examination* (BSE) beginning at age 20 and they should have their exam technique reviewed by their physician or provider. Women practicing BSE should perform their exams after their menstrual period when breasts are less congested.

A study of breast cancer patients sorted by the frequency of BSE found those who practiced monthly BSE presented with a lump averaging 2.1 cm, infrequent BSE averaged 2.5 cm and no BSE averaged 3.6 cm. The group who did monthly BSE also had fewer axillary nodes affected by cancer.

Between 80 and 95% of all breast cancers are discovered by the patient, then confirmed by the physician and mammography. It's been reasoned that if blind people can be taught to read Braille with their fingers, an individual has the capacity to be trained to detect small breast lumps. Because mortality is decreased with early detection, it's incumbent on both physicians and women to improve their skills in performing breast examinations.

There are a number of methods for practicing breast examination and studies have shown considerable variation in effectiveness at detecting lesions. Two scientists from the University of Florida, Dr. Henry S. Pennypacker and Dr. Mark Kane Goldstein initiated a research program to improve the accuracy of the clinical breast examination. They developed life-like silicone breast models imbedded with varying sizes of simulated tumors. They found that with training and practice, human fingers can reliably detect a 0.3 cm imbedded lump approximately 80% of the time. They incorporated varying levels of pressure and a more systematic process to ensure a more comprehensive exam.

This methodology has been incorporated into a teaching method called *MammaCare* that is being incorporated in various women's centers around the country. I became certified as a *MammaCare* clinical breast examiner to improve care to my patients and to teach them this technique so that they can do more accurate breast self-examinations.

Key Points About Breast Cancer & Other Hormone Related Cancers

1. More deaths occur from heart disease than the next 16 causes of death combined including diabetes, all cancers, AIDS and accidents.
2. A first pregnancy before age 25 protects against breast cancer.
3. Dense breasts on mammography increase risk of breast cancer.
4. Small breast cancers less than 2.1 cm (2.5 cm = 1 inch) have a lower mortality than large breast cancers.
5. Positive family history occurs in only 15-20% of women with breast cancer but is an indication for closer monitoring and possible genetic testing .
6. "Bad estrogen" byproducts increase risk of breast cancer, ovarian cancer and uterine cancer.
7. "Good estrogen" byproducts lower risk of breast cancer, ovarian cancer, and uterine cancer and lower the risk of heart disease.

You Can Lower Your Risk of Breast Cancer With the Following Actions

1. Lifestyle which includes exercise, not smoking and little or no alcohol

2. Diet which includes intake of cruciferous vegetables (broccoli, cauliflower, etc.) and low intake of saturated animal fats

3. Twenty to thirty minutes of midday sun exposure or vitamin D3 supplementation to maintain adequate 25-hydroxy vitamin D blood levels

4. Maintain a normal body weight

5. Sleep 7 to 8 hours nightly

6. Breast-feed your babies

7. Monthly self breast examinations after proper training from your physician

8. Monitor for "bad estrogen" and "good estrogen" byproducts under the guidance of your physician

Chapter 19

Breast Cancer

It's understandable that women fear breast cancer but hopefully you now have a better perspective of risks and ways to modify those risks. To make an intelligent decision about estrogen and breast cancer, you must first know the risk of breast cancer if you NEVER take estrogen. Denying yourself estrogen does not mean your risk of breast cancer is zero. According to 2005 statistics from the *National Institutes of Health*, among 10,000 women who never took HRT, 30 cases of breast cancer would be expected to occur in 5.2 years. If you compare that figure to 10,000 women who did take HRT, the number of cases of breast cancer increases to 38 cases. This is only an increase of eight cases in 10,000 women. This means if you take HRT for 5 years, you will get breast cancer 0.38% of the time versus 0.30% of the time if you don't take HRT, an increase of 0.08%. These statistics apply to women on all forms of HRT. More studies are needed to determine if different types of HRT are associated with varying risks of breast cancer.

Timing of Estrogen Initiation After Menopause - The "Gap Time Effect"

A 2006 study analyzed the effects of Premarin on the risk of breast cancer and showed no increase in breast cancer after 7.1 years. There was actually a trend toward a lower incidence of breast cancer that was totally unexpected. A possible explanation for this reduced risk in breast cancer from Premarin follows. It appears that the time when estrogen is first initiated after menopause affects breast cancer risk. Starting estrogen more than 5 years after onset of menopause is considered a long gap time while starting estrogen immediately after menopause is considered a short gap time. This is a complex issue so let me first give you some background to make it easier to understand.

Most invasive breast cancers are the end result of a decades-long evolution of increasingly abnormal premalignant cells. Estrogen is thought to promote breast cancer NOT by causing new cancer cells but rather by accelerating the growth of these small, premalignant cells so they become detectable on clinical exam or mammogram. When breast tissue is deprived of estrogen at menopause for many years, it can cause shrinkage of these premalignant cells. Recall that the WHI participants who started Premarin had been menopausal without estrogen for an average of 8 years.

A very interesting phenomenon has been observed in breast cancer cell cultures. When the cancer cells are deprived of estrogen for a long time, subsequent addition of estrogen paradoxically causes reduction in further growth of the breast cancer cells. In the 70s before the advent of estrogen blockers like tamoxifen, breast cancer was actually treated with high-dose synthetic estrogens. In a 2009 study, 66 breast cancer patients who had relapsed despite seven years of estrogen blockers, were treated with either high-dose or low-dose estrogen. After 24 weeks of treatment, tumors had shrunk or stopped growing in a third of both groups. This mechanism may explain the decrease in breast cancer seen in the women who took Premarin after having had no estrogen for eight years.

To evaluate the effect of a short gap time, the French E4N observational study analyzed incidence of breast cancer in newly menopausal women who were started on synthetic estrogen or estrogen and synthetic progestin within two years of menopause. They showed a 50% increase in breast cancer compared to women not taking hormones. This increased risk was not seen in newly menopausal women who were taking estradiol and progesterone. Women who waited three years after menopause to start synthetic estrogen or estrogen and synthetic progestin did not show this increased risk. Because synthetic hormones confer increased breast cancer risk when started soon after menopause, it appears safer to choose estradiol and progesterone.

Duration of estrogen use

While the increased risk of breast cancer from five years of hormone use is minimal, the risks increase with longer exposure to hormones. A collaborative reanalysis of data from 51 epidemiological studies of 52,705 women with breast cancer and 108,311 women without breast cancer estimated that for every 1000 women who take HRT for 10 or 15 years, there were 6 and 12 additional cases of breast cancer as compared to women on no HRT. That makes the increased risk at 10 and 15 years, 0.6% and 1.2%, respectively. The **Million Women Study** (MWS) is an observational study of women's health being conducted in the United Kingdom and represents the largest study of its kind in the world. In 2003, MWS published a study on breast cancer and reported a lower risk of breast cancer from topical HRT than oral HRT but the differences were not statistically significant. The magnitude of increased risk for breast cancer was greatest in the women on combined estrogen-progestin. See section on *Risks of Combined Estrogen-Progestins*. Increased risk of breast cancer normalizes within five years of stopping hormones.

Ovarian Cancer

A similar case can be made for ovarian cancer, another uncommon cancer which has been associated with HRT. In 2007, a Million Woman Study on ovarian cancer showed a rate of 2.6 cases of ovarian cancer per 1000 women on HRT, compared with 2.2 cases of ovarian cancer per 1000 women not taking HRT. So the excess risk from HRT was calculated at 0.4 cases per 1000. So, the risk of ovarian cancer from taking HRT for five years is 0.26% and without HRT the risk is 0.22% or one extra case of ovarian cancer in 2500 women. In the Danish study of 909,946 women followed for 8 years, the excess risk was 0.6 cases per 1000, but this was not considered statistically significant. So, essentially ovarian cancer is a rare disease that should not affect a woman's decision to take hormone therapy.

Endometrial Cancer (Uterine Cancer)

Obesity markedly increases the risk of endometrial cancer, because of the increased estrogen produced by fat cells. In a study of 495,477 women followed for 16 years, the most obese group had a 6.25 times higher risk of dying (not just being diagnosed) with endometrial cancer than those with normal weight. Obesity is also associated with endometrial cancer occurring in younger women (under age 45). In a study of 3580 obese women who went through menopause before the age of 45, those with a BMI of 30-34.9 had a similar six times increase in being diagnosed with cancer. However, those with a BMI over 35 had a greater than twenty times risk of being diagnosed with endometrial cancer.

Body mass index (BMI) is the most commonly used measurement for assessing obesity. To calculate your BMI, multiply your weight in pounds by 703, divide by height in inches

(5 feet=60 inches), and divide again by height in inches. A BMI of 18.5 to 24.9 is considered normal for most adults. A BMI of 30 is regarded as obesity and 40 or greater is morbid obesity.

It has been well established that for women with an intact uterus, taking estrogen without progesterone or a synthetic progestin carries an eight-fold increased risk of uterine cancer. However, giving estrogen in combination with either cyclic or continuous progesterone/progestin decreases this risk to less than the risk of women who never take HRT. When cyclic progestin is used for 10 or fewer days per month, risk of endometrial cancer is greater compared to using continuous daily progestin. Based on epidemiological data, it has been suggested that cyclic progestin should be used for 14 days of each month.

In an NIH study of 73,211 women, there was no increased risk of endometrial cancer in women who were treated with either estrogen with cyclic progestin for 10 to 14 days or estrogen with continuous progestin. The data establishes endometrial cancer is a risk that can be avoided. Women on HRT, with an intact uterus, should undergo a yearly *transvaginal ultrasound* (TVS) to ensure there is no excessive build-up of the endometrium, the lining of the uterus.

Women with an intact uterus who are on estrogen plus cyclic progesterone generally have a monthly period, which is easily manageable and predictable. They should not have very heavy or painful periods, or bleeding between periods. Such symptoms indicate they should undergo a TVS and possibly an endometrial biopsy or diagnostic hysteroscopy to determine the cause of the problem periods. A hysteroscopy is an office procedure that allows a gynecologist to visualize the inside of the uterus with a small scope containing a camera. If daily progesterone is given, most women will have irregular bleeding for the first three to six months. After six months, 75% of such women will stop all irregular bleeding. Those who continue irregular bleeding are advised to switch to cyclic progesterone.

With regard to cancers, because I'm an optimist, I choose to focus on the fact that if I decide to take HRT for five years, 99.62% of the time I will not get breast cancer and 99.74% of the time I will not get ovarian cancer. Even if I reach the age of 85 years when the risk of breast cancer is 1 in 8, I choose to focus on the probability of 7 in 8 that I won't get cancer. Provided progesterone/progestin is given appropriately and properly monitored, increase in the risk of endometrial cancer is substantially eliminated.

For myself, I have decided to take hormones for longer than five years. While my risk for breast cancer and ovarian cancer may be slightly increased, I believe the benefits of HRT and the resulting better quality of life outweigh the risks. However, I must reiterate that this is a very personal decision that each woman needs to make with her own physician based on her own unique situation and risk factors. Understanding the absolute numbers and how they interrelate, instead of just hearing sound bites of an "increased risk," enables you to make a more informed decision.

If you choose to take hormones for longer than five years, you are well advised to follow the lifestyle choices that lessen your risk: regular exercise, avoiding smoking and alcohol, and maintaining optimal body weight. Because aging is associated with a decline in muscle mass, especially in sedentary individuals, ideal weight is better assessed by measuring body composition of lean muscle and fat. Muscle stores can be maintained with a program of resistance weight training two to three times weekly.

Ideally, estrogen metabolism should be monitored and adjusted as needed to favorable levels. The following risks of HRT are less common or less serious but nonetheless can affect the quality of life for some women. I list them to make you aware of them so that you may address them with your physician.

1. Dry Eye Syndrome

This is a condition characterized by symptoms of burning or irritation of the eyes due to lack of tears. A cohort study in 25,655 menopausal women followed for 48 months showed that "estrogen only HRT" increased the risk of dry eye by 69%, and "combined estrogen plus progesterone/progestin HRT" increased the risk by only 29%. Women on no HRT had the same risk as premenopausal women. It's unclear whether this is related to the use of estrogen or to the lack of androgens that are commonly deficient in menopausal women. If androgen levels are deficient in these women on HRT, additional testosterone therapy might be indicated.

2. Raynaud's phenomenon

Raynaud's is a condition where the small blood vessels in the hands or feet respond to cold temperatures with vasospasm (a sudden constriction of a blood vessel). Deprived of oxygen, the skin turns blue then white and finally red when the blood flow resumes. In one study of 497 women from the Framingham Offspring Study, Raynaud's phenomenon occurred in 19.1% of menopausal women on estrogen alone. This effect seems to be related to giving estrogen alone since there was no increased occurrence reported in postmenopausal women on combined HRT or in those women on no HRT.

3. Bronchospasm and asthma

In the Nurses' Health Study of 36,094 menopausal women followed for 10 years, an increased incidence of new onset asthma was noted in women taking oral conjugated equine estrogens at doses higher than 0.625 mg. The studies on whether estrogen worsens airway function in women with asthma conflicting. One study showed a mild worsening while in another study, estrogen had no effect on negative airway function. The mechanism for any effect of estrogen on the bronchial airways is unclear.

Interestingly, estrogen has been shown to support the integrity of the alveoli, the tiny sacs in the lung where oxygen and carbon dioxide are exchanged. This explains the increased incidence of emphysema in women who don't take HRT. Therefore, there should be no concern in giving HRT to women with chronic obstructive pulmonary disease or emphysema.

4. Epilepsy

Women with epilepsy sometimes report a worsening of seizures that occurs right before a period or at ovulation. The medical term for this phenomenon is catamenial seizures. This is thought to be related to marked changes in estradiol that occurs at these times. Progesterone has a calming effect on the nervous system, and it is likely the drop in progesterone at the end of the cycle that explains the catamenial seizures.

A small study was done in 42 women to evaluate the effect of perimenopause and menopause on the course of epilepsy. Twenty-nine women had either no change or a decrease in seizures at menopause while 13 had an increase in seizures. Women who had catamenial seizures prior to menopause had increased occurrence in perimenopause but a decreased occurrence in menopause. In women with a history of catamenial seizures, HRT during perimenopause seemed to increase the risk of seizures. Since perimenopause is associated with more internal fluctuations of both estrogen and progesterone, perhaps such variance explains the increased occurence of seizures.

5. Systemic lupus erythematosus (SLE)

Systemic lupus erythematosus (SLE) is an autoimmune disease often treated with steroids or immunosuppressive drugs. These women may be more prone to premature menopause because of autoimmune ovarian failure or from the immunosuppressive drugs. In the Nurses' Health Study, with never users of HRT as the reference group, the natural incidence of this group developing SLE over the 14 years of the study was an age-adjusted relative risk of 2.1. Those women who took HRT over this same time period had a slightly higher age-adjusted relative risk of 2.5. However, SLE patients who took HRT tended to have improvement in SLE symptoms over time and it seemed to be independent of menopause. If flares occur with HRT, they tend to be mild.

6. Uterine Fibroids

Fibroids are benign uterine growths that can occur in premenopausal women. They are often estrogen driven but tend to resolve with the onset of menopause. Because of concerns that HRT could worsen fibroids, a systematic review of five randomized controlled trials found that HRT could cause fibroid growth, but this typically occurred without clinical symptoms. In a prospective three year study, fibroids grew in the first two years of HRT but by the third year of HRT, fibroids regressed to baseline sizes. Therefore, the presence of fibroids do not constitute a reason to avoid HRT.

7. Endometriosis

In postmenopausal women who had endometriosis prior to menopause, starting HRT may cause aggravation of endometriosis symptoms. Since the amount of prescribed hormones is much lower than levels produced naturally in younger women, I generally find that this issue is mild or easily managed by providing the right balance of estradiol, progesterone and testosterone. Women who have had a hysterectomy are not generally given progesterone. However, if such women are exhibiting endometriosis symptoms on estrogen alone, small doses of cyclic progesterone short-term may relieve symptoms from residual endometriosis.

8. Parkinson's disease

Men who regularly consume caffeine-containing drinks have a lower risk of *Parkinson's disease* (PD), but this association is not seen in women. In the Nurses' Health Study, 77,713 women were followed for 18 years and no difference in PD was seen in menopausal women with or without HRT. However, when these two groups were analyzed by caffeine intake, those women on HRT who consumed six or more cups of coffee daily had a fourfold higher risk of developing PD. The mechanism is unclear but suggests that women taking HRT should avoid such excessive intake of caffeine.

Chapter 20

Increased risks from oral estrogens

Many past studies showing risks have not compared the difference in risks between oral and topical estrogen administration. The studies have predominantly involved oral conjugated equine estrogens, because that is the most commonly prescribed hormone in the U.S. While 70% of French and Italian women use topical estradiol, only 15% of American women use topical therapy. American women predominantly use oral estrogen, with Premarin and Prempro being the most common form.

After any medicine is swallowed, it is absorbed by the digestive system and must be metabolized by the liver before it reaches the rest of the body. This aspect of drug metabolism is called the *"first-pass effect"* and often markedly reduces the amount of active drug distributed to the rest of the body. To compensate for this reduction, fairly large doses of oral estrogen must be given. For example, an oral dose of 1 milligram of oral estradiol must be given to achieve the same blood levels as *0.1 milligram* of topical estradiol. The *"first pass effect"* from oral estrogen also causes the liver to produce harmful proteins, clotting factors, and proinflammatory substances that contribute to the following problems.

Weight Gain

Many woman are concerned about their weight. Estradiol deficiency at menopause leads to a thickening around the waist caused by visceral obesity. *Visceral obesity* is the medical term for this fat around your middle and it includes increased fat in vital organs like the heart, kidneys, and the liver. This increased fat mass leads to an increase in a hormone called leptin that is produced by fat cells. Topical, but not oral, estradiol appears to prevent this increase in body fat and leptin.

Studies also show that oral estrogen increases the production of *thyroxine-binding globulin* (TBG), the carrier protein for thyroid hormone. Higher levels of TBG lower the level of available thyroid hormone thereby lowering metabolic rate. All these changes explain a common complaint I hear from women who have been on oral estrogen, *"After starting oral estrogen I put on 15 pounds in the first month and I didn't increase my calories or lower my exercise. Now I'm eating less and exercising more, and I just keep gaining!"*

Insulin-like growth factor (IGF-1), an indicator of growth hormone production, conserves muscle stores. Oral estrogen suppresses IGF-1 and this is another mechanism for increased fat and loss of muscle. Oral estrogen is associated with a decreased ability to burn fat that contributes to increased fat stores. While several studies have shown an improved muscle:fat mass ratio from topical estrogen, there is still not universal agreement. The majority of studies showing no increased fat or decreased muscle from oral estrogen were in women who were not overweight or obese when they started oral estrogen.

Sexual Dysfunction

Oral estrogen, but not topical estrogen increases *sex hormone binding globulin* (SHBG) by greater than 100%. SHBG is the carrier protein in the blood that binds estrogen and testosterone. High SHBG levels reduce the amount of circulating estrogen and testosterone that can lead to sexual dysfunction. In addition, blood levels of oral estrogen peak at 4 to 5 hours and are not measurable by 8 to 10 hours. Lower estrogen and testosterone for 10 hours and no hormones for 14 hours each day leads to atrophy of genital tissues. This explains why these women may develop vaginal dryness and painful intercourse. No matter how much you love your partner, if your brain receives pain signals every time you have intercourse, this will definitely dampen your sex drive.

I have had women tell me, *"When I have sex, it feels like torture, and I always bleed afterwards."* When a woman starts avoiding sex, this may lead to marital strife because her husband may feel she no longer loves him. I've seen many marriages derailed when a woman goes through menopause and develops these symptoms. The good news is that by changing to topical estrogen and utilizing vaginal estrogen, these problems are almost always corrected.

Heart Disease, Ischemic Strokes and Blood clots

Increased heart disease from oral estrogen was seen only in WHI women who started HRT more than 20 years after menopause. A 2007 reanalysis of the WHI data by age and years since menopause showed that women who started either Premarin or Prempro within 10 years of menopause had no statistically significant increase or decrease in risk of heart disease. (This essentially translates to no protective benefit against heart disease.)

In September 2008, an observational study of 698,098 Danish women reported the risk of heart attack is affected by the type of HRT and the route of administration. **The women on oral estrogen had no reduction in the risk of heart attacks when compared to women who took no HRT. However, women** receiving topical estradiol therapy had 38% fewer heart attacks compared to women who did not take HRT suggesting that topical estradiol can reduce the incidence of heart disease.

Metabolic syndrome (MBS) is a cardiac condition diagnosed when three or more of the following five risk factors are present: a waist measurement of 35 inches or more for women and 40 inches or more for men; an elevated triglyceride level; a low HDL cholesterol level; a blood pressure greater than 130/85; or a fasting blood sugar of 100 or greater. In a study of obese postmenopausal women with MBS, oral but not topical estrogen increased the levels of matrix metalloproteinase (MMP-9) , a harmful pro-inflammatory protein.

Standard dose oral HRT increases the stroke risk by one third in otherwise healthy postmenopausal women. In a large cohort study of 75,668 women, oral estrogen in both low and high doses was associated with increased risk of stroke. Topical estradiol in daily doses of 0.05 mg or less had no increased risks of stroke.

Oral estrogen has been associated with a two to four-fold increased risk of blood clots in the lower legs. This risk is further increased by greater age, obesity, surgery, and long periods of immobilization (e.g. long plane or automobile ride.) If the clot remains in the leg, it is commonly knows as "phlebitis," which means inflammation of a vein resulting in localized pain and irritation. The medical term is thrombophlebitis. If it involves superficial veins on the skin surface it usually resolves quickly with proper care. If the clot occurs in larger deep veins, this requires medical evaluation. The blood clot may break off and travel to the lungs causing a potentially life-threatening condition called pulmonary embolism.

Oral estrogen increases triglycerides and the "bad" choles-terol known as *low density lipoprotein* (LDL). LDL is a primary cholesterol component that contributes to heart disease and strokes. While oral estrogen has been shown to also increase the "good" cholesterol known as *high density lipoprotein*, (HDL), this increase has not been associated with a corre-sponding reduction in cardiovascular risk. A possible expla-nation is that oral estrogen also increases harmful pro-in-flammatory proteins in the blood including *C-reactive protein* (CRP) and MMP-9. Since chronic inflammation leads to heart disease and strokes, anything which increases inflammation can worsen these diseases.

An important role of HDL is to keep your arteries clean. It does this by circulating throughout your blood vessels pick-ing up cellular debris and harmful products. Another reason for the lack of benefit from increased HDL was seen in a 2004 study that showed that oral but not topical, estrogen increases *serum amyloid A* (SAA), a harmful protein which needs to be cleared by HDL. The increased SAA increases the workload of HDL, and thereby reduces the heart-protective and antioxi-dant capacity of HDL. Oral estrogen also increases clotting factors including fibrinogen, Factor VII and antithrombin III that thicken the blood and make it easier to form clots leading to heart disease and strokes.

Oral estrogen causes decreases in *insulin growth factor-1* (IGF-1), an indicator of growth hormone production. Lower levels of IGF-1 or estradiol lead to increased thickening of the inner two layers of the carotid arteries (the intima and me-dia.) A *Carotid Intima-Media Thickening* (CIMT) test, a nonin-vasive ultrasound measurement of these layers, is done yearly to monitor a patient's risk for heart disease or strokes. Lower levels of IGF-1 can lead to a loss of muscle and an increase in visceral obesity.

Visceral obesity is the medical term for increased fat deposits in vital organs such as the heart, liver and kidneys. The typical individual with visceral obesity will have a pot belly and fairly normal arms and legs. We call this body type the "apple" shape rather than a "pear" which is more typical of the female form. Even women who are normal weight and take oral estrogen may notice that their fat has shifted, and they have increased thickening around their waist.

Insulin is a hormone essential to life and its actions demonstrates the importance of homeostasis or optimal balance. Without insulin you die in a matter of days as can occur in type-1 diabetics. On the other hand, excess insulin levels cause you to age prematurely. This tendency to excess insulin levels is called *insulin resistance* and can occur with aging. It is a serious risk factor that leads to higher risks of heart disease and stroke. Oral estrogen, but not topical estrogen, further increases the risk of insulin resistance. Oral estrogen also results in elevated leptin levels that further contribute to insulin resistance and visceral obesity.

A *meta-analysis* is a statistical summary that combines data from multiple clinical studies. By increasing the number of study patients, one is better able to see trends and draw conclusions. A French meta-analysis of seventeen studies, *showed oral HRT doubles or triples the risk of clots while topical HRT showed no increased risk of clots.*

Gallbladder Disease and Surgery

Treatment with oral estrogen or oral estrogen/progestin increases the risk of cholecystitis (inflammation of the gallbladder), gallstones, and surgery to remove the gallbladder. In a reanalysis of WHI, the WHI investigators found the annual incidence of gallstones in women on PremPro over 5.6 years was 55 per 10,000 person years as compared to 35 in those not on HRT.

The incidence of gallstones in women on Premarin only was 78 per 10,000 person years as compared to 47 per 10,000 person years in those women not on HRT. A person year is a statistical measure representing the sum of the number of years that each study participant was treated with a drug.

A large study of women ages 50 to 69 in the United Kingdom showed a higher risk of gallbladder disease with oral than with topical estrogen. It also showed that Premarin and Prempro had slightly higher risks than oral estradiol and that high doses of estrogen had a higher risk than low doses of estrogen. Ten years after stopping estrogen, gallbladder disease decreased but minimal increased risk persisted.

Migraine Headaches

Oral estrogen can increase platelet aggregation that may worsen migraines. In addition, fluctuations in estradiol levels from the once-a-day flooding of the liver by oral estrogens may trigger migraine headaches. Topical estrogen provides more consistent estradiol blood levels.

KEY POINTS:

Use of Oral Estrogen Increases Risks For Following Conditions:

1. Weight Gain, especially around the waist
2. Sexual Dysfunction
3. Heart Disease in Women Starting HRT 10 Years after Menopause
4. Blood clots and Strokes
5. Gallstones
6. Migraines

In summary, all these adverse affects can be greatly reduced by choosing topical estradiol over oral estrogen, and I see no justification for prescribing oral estrogen.

Chapter 21

*Increased risks of adding daily oral
synthetic progestins to oral estrogens*

Continuous combined oral HRT is the combination of a daily dose of an oral estrogen and an oral progestin. They are commonly formulated into one tablet for patient convenience. **All the risks previously mentioned for oral estrogen also apply to these combined oral estrogen/progestin products.** Prempro is an example of this type of therapy and is commonly used in the US. There are many other commercially available formulations that combine an oral estrogen and an oral synthetic progestin (*FemHRT, Activella* and *Angeliq*).

This regimen is often used because most women who still have their uterus will stop having any menstrual bleeding within six months of continuous use. While women like not having periods, this convenience may lead to serious consequences. Giving progestin every day defies the basic physiology of the body, because in healthy premenopausal women, progesterone is only produced for two weeks each month. Several studies have shown that adding a continuous daily synthetic progestin to estrogen decreases the beneficial actions of estrogen. Whether using daily progesterone has the same detrimental effect is less clear since most of the studies have been done with the more commonly used synthetic progestins. Some women have a psychological aversion to the notion of having a menstrual period again even though they are very light and easily manageable. If this is an issue, then we opt for continuous daily progesterone.

Progestins Reduce The Cardiac Benefits of Estrogen

All the adverse effects from the oral route of administration of estrogen as previously outlined can also occur from oral Prempro. However, the addition of the progestin seems to confer additional cardiac risk. Perhaps giving progestins daily instead of in cycles of 14 days each calendar month may be a factor in this increased risk. Earlier observational studies, like the Nurses' Health Study, predominantly used oral cyclic progestins and did not show an increased risk of heart disease.

While estrogen increases the beneficial HDL cholesterol, adding a continuous synthetic oral progestin lowers HDL by 8 to 18%. Addition of oral, micronized progesterone causes little or no adverse effects on HDL. An animal study showed that adding MPA to estradiol blocks the conversion of estradiol to an important beneficial byproduct made in the liver called 2-methoxyestradiol.

In the Women's Health Initiative, a randomized, placebo-controlled trial showed no change in the incidence of heart disease in women starting Prempro within 10 years of menopause when compared with placebo. Women starting Prempro 10 years after menopause had an increased risk of heart disease which increased the more time had elapsed since menopause.

The 2009 Danish Study, an observational study of 698,098 women, found those who took continuous combined oral HRT had a 35% increased risk of heart attacks compared to women who did not take hormones. In the women taking topical estradiol plus cyclic progesterone or cyclic progestin, there were 38% fewer heart attacks.

I had an acquaintance, Janet, who became newly menopausal and was exhibiting the typical symptoms. Her physician promptly started her on a daily combination pill containing synthetic estrogen and progestin. Within days of starting that therapy, she developed new-onset chest pain sending her to the emergency room (ER). At the ER, Janet was evaluated and sent home and referred to a cardiologist who did stress testing and told her everything was normal. When she continued to have intermittent chest pain, her physician changed her to a combined topical estradiol/synthetic progestin patch. The pain lessened but she still had occasional chest pain. Not until she was finally put on topical estradiol with cyclic oral progesterone did she finally have resolution of her chest discomfort. Imagine the cost savings and the angst that would have been avoided if she had just been put on topical estradiol and cyclic progesterone from the beginning!

Progestins Increase Blood Clots in Veins & Pulmonary Emboli

Blood clots in veins in the lower legs can occur with aging and obesity, especially after prolonged inactivity like sitting in a car or plane for many hours. While Premarin can cause an increase in clots, the addition of the progestin in Prempro, leads to an even greater risk of blood clots in the legs.

Oral estrogen/progestin combination drugs cause increased production of clotting factors by the liver through the *"first-pass effect"*. A unique feature of these blood clots is they can become dislodged from arteries in the lower legs, travel through the circulatory system, and cause a pulmonary embolus (blockage of a pulmonary artery), a serious, potentially fatal condition.

Progestins Increase Breast Cancer Risk

Addition of progestins increases mammographic density, a risk factor associated with an increased risk of breast cancer. Another harmful effect of daily synthetic progestin is to turn off apoptosis, a natural defense mechanism of the body that destroys early cancer cells. This inhibition of apoptosis has been demonstrated in cultures of cells from both normal and breast cancer tissues. Inhibition of apoptosis by medroxyprogesterone, a synthetic progestin, has been demonstrated in cultures of cells from both normal and breast cancer tissues.

A 2010 study published in *Nature* has uncovered how synthetic progestins like MPA increase the risk of breast cancer. MPA triggers increased production of a protein molecule RANKL, which is essential to regulation of bone mass and is also involved in milk production. The increased RANKL in breast cells, causes these breast cells to divide and multiply and fail to die when they should. Moreover, stem cells in the breast become able to regenerate, ultimately resulting in breast cancer.

MPA is marketed as Provera and in combination with Premarin as Prempro, the drugs used in the WHI study. MPA is also found in long-acting injectable contraceptive, including Depo-Provera which is given every three months. Numerous studies analyzing breast cancer risk by the type of HRT have shown the addition of a synthetic progestin confers an increased risk of breast cancer and increased mortality from the breast cancer.

In a 2002 study of 3823 women followed for five years, women on continuous combined HRT had an increased breast cancer risk while women on HRT with cyclic progestin or estrogen only had no increased risk of breast cancer. A 2002 French study in 3175 women using topical estrogen therapy with cyclic progesterone for 8.9 years showed no increased incidence of breast cancer.

The *Million Women Study* published in 2003 studied the incidence of breast cancer in women ages 50 to 64 followed for five years. Current users of HRT had a higher risk of developing breast cancer. When analyzed by the type of HRT, women on estrogen only had a relative risk of 1.30 while the estrogen-progestin group had a much higher relative risk of 2.00. When analyzed by the route of delivery, topical estrogen tended to have the lowest relative risk at 1.24, oral estrogen intermediate at 1.32 and estrogen implants were the highest at 1.65. However, these differences were not considered to be statistically significant. This study showed no difference in risk between cyclic and continuous progestin/progesterone regimens.

A *meta-analysis* combines data from multiple independent studies to determine the risk of a particular problem in certain populations. In 2005, Collins did a meta-analysis of 22 studies involving more than 1.5 million women to determine the risk of breast cancer in postmenopausal women taking estrogen or estrogen-progestin. His analysis showed breast cancer risk is increased more with estrogen-progestin than with estrogen alone. A small difference of less breast cancer risk was seen in women on cyclic progestin compared to those on continuous progestin. Women normalized the risk of breast cancer within 5 years of stopping hormone use.

A *prospective cohort* is a type of observational study in which similar individuals (e.g. menopausal women of a certain age) are followed for a number of years to determine the effects of different medications or lifestyle habits on various risks.

The 2007 E3N-EPIC study, is a prospective cohort French study of 80,377 post-menopausal women followed for 12 years to assess the risks among different forms of HRT. The study reported increased risk of breast cancer with the use of oral estrogen plus synthetic progestins or with the use of oral estrogen alone as compared to women on no HRT. Those women taking topical estradiol plus daily progesterone had no increased risk of breast cancer as compared to women who never used HRT. **This study supports the idea that bioidentical hormones are safer than synthetics, especially for progesterone versus synthetic progestins.**

Women Smokers with Lung cancer on Combined HRT May have Decreased Survival

Large *observational studies* have shown HRT offers protection from the risk of lung cancer. In a study of 422 women with lung cancer, those who had previously undergone bilateral removal of ovaries had a significantly higher risk of developing lung cancer. Women who had their ovaries removed had a higher risk of lung cancer than women who went through natural menopause. Numerous studies, including WHI, have shown that HRT is not associated with an increased risk of lung cancer. However, a 2009 reanalysis of the WHI study showed that women with lung cancer on HRT had a decreased survival rate as compared to those on no HRT. A study of 498 women with lung cancer on HRT showed decreased survival rates in women on HRT but this finding was statistically significant only in those women on HRT who were smokers. Another study of 397 women with lung cancer who were mostly smokers showed no difference in survival between groups on HRT and no HRT.

An interesting study showed that progesterone receptors are present in about half of lung tumors. Progesterone mediates pathways that induce apoptosis (programmed cell death) in lung cancer cells and reduces lung tumor growth. It has been suggested that if progesterone receptors are present in lung tumors, progesterone could inhibit lung tumor growth. This could present a potential, new therapeutic weapon for treating lung cancer.

Because of the questions raised by these studies, the ultimate decision to continue HRT in a woman with lung cancer needs to be made in careful consultation with the treating oncologist. If the decision is made to continue HRT, it appears prudent to choose estradiol and cyclic progesterone over combined estrogen-progestin.

Progestins Increase Dementia & Cognitive Dysfunction

Most large studies of combined estrogen with continuous progestin show no benefit of HRT in preserving cognitive function or preventing dementia compared to those on no HRT. A few small studies have shown a modest benefit in cognition from oral estrogen but worsening of cognition from oral combined estrogen/synthetic progestins. The *Women's Health Initiative Memory Study* (WHIMS), an ancillary study of the WHI using combined estrogen/synthetic progestins, showed an increased risk of dementia (40 cases in 2229 women on HRT compared to 21 cases in women on no HRT).

Since estrogen alone is known to protect brain cells, it is possible the increased dementia that occurred in WHIMS resulted from the addition of a continuous synthetic progestin to the estrogen. Such an effect has been demonstrated in a laboratory study of neuronal brain cells subjected to toxic chemicals.

Providing estradiol and progesterone to the brain cells protected the brain neurons against cell death. However, when *MPA* (synthetic progestin) was added to the culture medium, the protective effects of estradiol were blocked.

A *positron emission tomography* (PET) scan is a diagnostic imaging scan that uses low-dose radioactive sugar to measure functional brain activity. PET scans can be used to demonstrate patterns associated with Alzheimer's disease. In a 2010 study, 53 postmenopausal women at increased risk for Alzheimer's disease and previously on estrogen at least a year underwent a baseline PET scan. Women taking estradiol performed three standard deviations higher in verbal memory than women taking Premarin. Women taking an estrogen/progestin combination pill (Prempro) had lower brain metabolism than women taking estrogen alone.

The *Cache County Study on Memory, Health and Aging* has been following a group of 5092 seniors since 1995 and reported that HRT was associated with a reduction in *Alzheimer's disease* (AD) by approximately one-half. Whereas AD risk in females over age 80 was twice that of males, the risk in females using HRT for longer than 10 years dropped to levels seen in males. HRT was also associated with better cognitive performance in those without dementia.

A few small studies show topical estrogen positively influences postmenopausal memory and may offer some protective effect against the cognitive decline seen in Alzheimer's. When large-scale studies comparing the different benefits and risks according to the type of HRT are done, it should provide helpful guidelines on which HRT is the safest and most effective.

Progestins Increase Incontinence

Stress incontinence is the medical term for involuntary leakage of urine that occurs when a woman sneezes or coughs or with increased exercise. With urge incontinence, a woman can have involuntary leakage of urine if she does not get to the bathroom quickly enough. This causes her to urinate frequently and she may have repeated urination as often as every 30 minutes to an hour. This latter type of incontinence is similar to the urgency most women have when they have a bladder infection but it occurs in the absence of infection.

For years, HRT was felt to be beneficial in preventing and treating urinary incontinence. However, in the 2001 *Heart and Estrogen/Progestin Replacement Study* (HERS), oral conjugated estrogens plus medroxyprogesterone (Prempro) increased both stress and urge incontinence within four months of starting therapy. Association of urinary incontinence with oral estrogen and estrogen/progestin was also seen in the Nurses' Health Study II, a study of 7341 postmenopausal women ages 37 to 54. The WHI study reported that women who were continent at the start of the study had an increased risk of both stress and urge incontinence after one year on either oral Premarin or Prempro. Those with pre-existing incontinence developed worsening of their condition with either medication.

One study using ultra low-dose topical estradiol showed no worsening of incontinence. In my own clinical experience using topical estradiol in over 100,000 female patient visits, I have not seen a worsening of incontinence with topical estrogen. However, I have seen women with preexisting incontinence who did not improve on topical estradiol until they were further treated with a course of vaginal estrogen.

Progestins Increase Hearing Loss

Estrogen HRT appears to delay hearing loss. However, the addition of a continuous progestin to estrogen appears to negatively affect hearing. Hearing abilities were analyzed in a group of 124 women ages 60 to 86 taking HRT, treated with estrogen + progestin (32), estrogen alone (30) and no HRT (62). The women underwent sophisticated hearing tests that evaluated both the peripheral (ear) and central (brain) auditory systems. One of the tests, the *hearing-in-noise test* (HINT) measures speech perception in background noise, the major complaint of hearing-impaired persons. The women receiving *estrogen + progestin* had poorer hearing abilities in both their peripheral and central auditory systems. The E+P group also showed more interference with perception of speech in background noise.

KEY POINTS:

Continuous Combined Oral Estrogen/Progestins increases risks for the following:

1. Heart Disease in women starting on HRT 10 years past menopause
2. Strokes
3. Blood Clots in Legs
4. Pulmonary Emboli
5. Breast Cancer
6. Dementia and Cognitive Decline
7. Urinary Incontinence
8. Hearing Loss

Based upon the current database, published clinical studies and my years of clinical experience, postmenopausal women who decide to take HRT and want to optimize benefits and lessen risks should opt for topical over oral estradiol and progesterone over a synthetic progestin. In women with a uterus who require the addition of progesterone, some but not all studies show a benefit from cyclic over continuous-use of progesterone/progestin.

Chapter 22

Since 2002, there has been intense focus on the increased risks associated with women taking estrogen therapy. I believe it is equally important to discuss and understand the consequences of NOT taking estrogen. Low estrogen can result in a breakdown and deterioration of the body and its systems. While you may not experience all of these effects without supplemental estrogen, you need to know about them so you can make an informed decision. Because estrogen reduces the risk of osteoporosis, heart disease, or Alzheimer's disease, this should be taken into consideration if you have a strong family history of these diseases.

Risks from estrogen in women who take HRT are often obscured because many older studies did not analyze the data based on the type of HRT given. Rather all the estrogen users were lumped into one group regardless of delivery system or use of a continuous/cyclic progestin.

Quality of Life

A low estrogen state contributes to a myriad of quality-of-life symptoms affecting your well-being which includes weight gain, insomnia, brain fog, heat intolerance/hot flashes, anxiety and irritability, crying for no reason, angry outbursts out of character for that person, fluid retention, body aches, stiffness and joint/muscle pains, constipation, frequent urination, dizziness, and fatigue. Women who had been adept at multi-tasking and juggling personal, family, and business duties suddenly find themselves feeling overwhelmed. Such symptoms can seriously impact productivity and relationships with family and friends. Some women may experience all or just a few of these symptoms.

Each woman is uniquely different in how she responds to a low-estrogen state. A few of these low estrogen symptoms like hot flashes may resolve over time even without ever taking HRT. Many symptoms can be alleviated with multiple medications. Restoring therapeutic estradiol levels does not necessarily mean that each symptom is 100% resolved because some of these symptoms may be multi-factorial. However, most of them can be improved with the proper dose of HRT.

QUALITY-OF-LIFE SYMPTOMS OF ESTROGEN DEFICIENCY

Increased Occurrence of the Following Symptoms:

1. Weight Gain, Especially Around the Waist
2. Fatigue
3. Insomnia
4. Heat Intolerance & Hot Flashes
5. Fluid Retention
6. Brain Fog
7. Anxiety & Irritability
8. "Weepies"
9. Feeling Overwhelmed
10. Body Aches, Stiffness and Joint/Muscle Pains
11. Itchy, flaky, thinning skin
12. Frequent urination
13. Constipation
14. Dizziness

SOME MEDICAL RISKS OF NOT TAKING ESTROGEN

More Occurrence of the Following:

1. Sexual Dysfunction
2. Hair Loss and Facial Hair
3. Premature Wrinkling, Thinning and Dry Skin
4. Urinary and/or Fecal Incontinence
5. Urinary Tract Infections, Vaginitis and Yeast Infections
6. Depression and Anxiety
7. Loss of Teeth and Poor Oral Health
8. Loss of Vision or Hearing
9. Heart Disease
10. Strokes
11. Decreased Memory & Mental function
12. Alzheimer's Disease
13. Osteoporosis
14. Diabetes
15. Colon Cancer
16. Reduced Lung Function
17. Osteoarthritis
18. Falls
19. Gout
20. Increased Mortality

Sexual Dysfunction

Without estrogen, many women start to have decreased libido and vaginal dryness. The vaginal dryness develops into vaginal atrophy. This makes sexual activity uncomfortable and can be disruptive to an otherwise healthy relationship. Painful intercourse affects 8 to 30% of menopausal women who are not on HRT. Most women also notice greater difficulty achieving orgasm.

Sexual function is a complex issue in women. Unlike men in whom libido directly correlates to the level of free testosterone, simply adding testosterone therapy does not always improve women's sexual function. A woman has to be in a healthy relationship where she perceives a level of trust and caring. Topical testosterone in physiological doses can increase desire, arousal, responsiveness and orgasm especially when combined with the right balance of estradiol since deficiencies in either hormone can contribute to sexual dysfunction.

Sexual intimacy is an important part of a healthy relationship, and I have seen many marriages derailed when the woman goes through perimenopause or menopause. When hormone levels drop and intercourse is painful, it is understandable that a woman develops decreased libido, no matter how much she may want to be with her partner. When his wife loses interest in sex, a husband can mistakenly think she no longer loves him, and he may reduce other forms of intimacy. Of course, HRT can't repair a bad marriage, but when sexual intimacy is restored between two people who love each other, it goes a long way towards healing their marriage. One patient's husband sent me a dozen roses after the HRT I prescribed for his wife restored their sexual relations.

Hair Loss and Facial Hair

Menopausal women without estrogen may lose hair on their head while developing an increase in facial or body hair. This hair loss is called androgenic alopecia and typically involves hair loss in the temples and crown of the head. When a woman's estrogen level remains low, the pituitary increases production of *follicle stimulating hormone* (FSH). FSH is the pituitary messenger hormone that signals the ovaries to produce more estrogen. Because there are no more eggs to produce estrogen,

FSH levels continue to rise and the high FSH serves as a marker of ovarian failure. Menopause is typically diagnosed with a high FSH and a low estrogen. High FSH stimulates other cells in the ovaries to increase testosterone production. The adrenal glands can also produce small amounts of testosterone.

Although this increase in testosterone is fairly modest, since there is no estrogen to offset it, it results in a mild type of male pattern hair loss. While they are losing hair from their scalp, postmenopausal women often experience an increase in facial hair from the increased testosterone. It is common to see menopausal women on no HRT with whiskers on their chin. Acne may also result from the hormone imbalance. This symptom does not have serious health consequences but a full head of hair is a socially regarded sign of femininity. Women are very distressed when they have a significant loss of scalp hair.

Premature Wrinkling, Thinning & Dry skin

Women often complain of itchy skin and scalp when their estrogen is low. When I see an older woman, I can usually tell if she is taking estrogen by looking at her skin. Estrogen is essential for preserving thickness and collagen content in the skin. Estrogen stimulates the release of transforming growth factor-beta that accelerates wound healing. With the loss of estrogen comes premature wrinkling and sagging of the skin. While this is not a serious health consequence, every woman likes to look her best as long as possible. When a woman starts estrogen, at her next visit, she usually tells me that her skin feels softer.

Increased Urinary and/or Fecal Incontinence

Lack of estrogen leads to atrophy and irritation of the tissues in the urethra and contributes to stress and urge incontinence. Women with a history of multiple or difficult vaginal deliveries may have had damage to nerves or muscles in the bladder and rectum, and this puts them at increased risk of incontinence. They may develop structural problems like prolapse of the uterus or bladder, rectocele, or cystocele. Without estrogen, these women tend to develop urinary incontinence and frequent urination. They must sometimes deal with the embarrassing loss of bladder control and resort to wearing pads. If the woman has had childbirth injury to the rectum, she may have fecal incontinence, which can be even more disturbing.

There are very effective hormone protocols, utilizing vaginal estrogen, that often improve these symptoms. Since oral estrogen or combined oral estrogen-synthetic progestin have been shown to worsen incontinence, systemic estrogen therapy should be given with topical estradiol.

A fairly new specialty called urogynecology deals with these problems. Urogynecologists must first complete a residency in obstetrics and gynecology or urology followed by a three-year fellowship in urogynecology. Most urogynecologists offer office-based physical therapy programs, which can be helpful with these problems. Surgery is sometimes required for women who do not respond to hormones and rehabilitation programs, especially if there is a structural problem.

Urinary Tract Infections, Atrophic Vaginitis, Yeast Infections

Lack of estrogen results in thinning of vaginal and urethral tissues and decreased vaginal secretions. These changes make the tissues more fragile and susceptible to irritation and recurrent urinary tract infections. In a trial of women with recurrent urinary tract infections, vaginal estrogen therapy was associated with a much greater likelihood of remaining free of infection. The group receiving estrogen experienced 0.5 infections per year as compared to 5.9 episodes per year in the group on placebo. In the HERS study, Prempro (oral conjugated equine estrogens combined with synthetic progestin) did not reduce the incidence of urinary tract infections compared to placebo.

Low estrogen also results in an increase in vaginal pH that changes the vaginal flora predisposing to vaginal yeast infections. The change in the vaginal tissues results in a condition called atrophic vaginitis that is characterized by irritation, itching and burning. While oral combined estrogen/progestin are not effective, all of these conditions are usually responsive to hormone regimens that utilize vaginal estrogen.

Depression & Mood

Estrogen deficiency has long been associated with increased mood symptoms and depression. However, patients are now more frequently diagnosed with depression because the widespread availability of prescription antidepressants has increased awareness among physicians and patients. A 2007 study by the *US Center for Disease Control and Prevention* showed that antidepressants are the most commonly prescribed prescription drugs. While these drugs offer an important therapeutic tool, restoring estrogen levels can sometimes avoid the need for antidepressants.

A *meta-analysis* of 26 studies evaluating the effects of HRT on perimenopausal and postmenopausal women showed lower levels of depression in hormone treated patients compared to those on placebo. The HERS study, a randomized, placebo-controlled double-blind trial of 2763 postmenopausal women with heart disease, showed that women with flushing assigned to HRT had improved mental health and less depression than those assigned to placebo.

A *randomized controlled study* in postmenopausal women showed improvement in mood and depression scores even in women who had no obvious menopausal symptoms. A study of 50 perimenopausal women with major depression, dysthymia or minor depression showed resolution of depression in 68% of those treated with 0.1 mg of topical estradiol for 12 weeks as compared to a 20% response in those women on no HRT. A study of 666 women who underwent surgical menopause on no HRT showed an increased long-term risk of depressive and anxiety symptoms.

Loss of Teeth and Poor Oral Health

Estrogen deficiency leads to dental problems including decreased saliva, decreased taste, oral discomfort, dryness, and increased dental cavities. Normal saliva contains digestive enzymes and antibacterial immune factors that contribute to oral health. Forty-four percent of postmenopausal women over 55 have periodontitis or gum disease often leading to tooth loss which can lead to implants or the need for dentures. In addition, estrogen has been shown to preserve facial bones, particularly the alveolar bone, which surrounds the teeth, reducing the likelihood of tooth loss.

Vision Loss, Age-Related Macular Degeneration and Cataracts

Age-related macular degeneration (AMD) gradually destroys a tiny part of the retina of the eye called the macula, needed for sharp, central vision. AMD is the leading cause of vision loss and blindness among older adults. The Nurses' Health Study of 74,996 women showed those women currently using HRT had a 48% lower risk for neovascular AMD, a late-stage form of AMD compared to women on no HRT. The WHI study also showed a lower risk of neovascular AMD in women on HRT as compared to the women on placebo.

A cataract is caused by clouding of the lens of the eye and can lead to poor vision or blindness. It can be corrected with surgical removal of the cataract. Before menopause the prevalence of cataracts is similar in males and females. After menopause, the prevalence of cataracts in females increases over men of equivalent age. One study of women with early-onset menopause, on no HRT, showed a 2.9 times increase in cataracts compared to women on HRT. In the *Framingham Heart Study*, postmenopausal women on HRT for 10 years or longer had a 60% reduction in cataracts compared with nonusers. In another study, cataracts were decreased by 70 to 80% in women on HRT compared with nonusers.

Hearing Loss

Without estrogen, the cochlea in the inner ear undergoes loss of minerals, decreased blood flow and loss of nerve cells leading to hearing loss. Estrogen HRT protects against this age-related decline in hearing. However, this protective effect can be diminished by addition of continuous synthetic progestin.

Turner's syndrome, a genetic condition associated with non-functioning ovaries, results in a low estrogen state. About 60% of Turner's women develop hearing loss that is thought to be related to their low estrogen state. A 35-year-old untreated Turner's patient will have hearing loss comparable to a 70-year-old woman. Women treated with drugs which block the actions of estradiol, like *Tamoxifen,* used as cancer therapy, can also develop hearing loss from the low estrogen state.

Heart Disease and Strokes

Heart disease and ischemic strokes were the number one and two causes of death in American women in 2006. Heart disease is responsible for half of all deaths of women over age 50. Menopausal women not on estrogen suffer increased heart disease. Observational studies have shown 40 to 60% less heart disease in women taking estrogen. Animal studies in monkeys have shown estrogen initiated at the time of menopause offers a 70% reduction in cardiovascular disease.

Strokes increase with age and women who undergo premature menopause without HRT have an increased risk of ischemic strokes. Animal studies show decreased ischemic stroke when estrogen is initiated at the onset of menopause. (Hemorrhagic stroke, caused by the sudden rupture of a weak blood vessel in the brain is much less common.)

Loss of estrogen leads to a decrease in beneficial HDL, increase in harmful LDL, increase in platelet aggregation, and increased overgrowth of cells in the arteries, all of which contribute to an increased risk of heart disease and strokes. The loss of estrogen at menopause also causes an increase in fibrinogen, a substance in the blood that causes clots. Increased fibrinogen leads to more heart disease and strokes.

Estrogen has anti-inflammatory effects on blood vessels and when deficient can lead to an increase in C-reactive protein that contributes to chronic inflammation. Because estrogen provides beneficial dilation of blood vessels, when levels are deficient, blood pressure rises and leads to an increased incidence of hypertension. Seventy-five percent of postmenopausal women develop hypertension which worsens heart disease. Premeno-pausal women consistently exhibit less heart disease than their male counterparts. At menopause, without estrogen, women's incidence of heart disease rapidly approaches that of men and worsens with increasing age.

Insulin is an important hormone required for utilization of glucose. When women become estrogen-deficient, they develop increased abdominal fat. The medical term for this abdominal fat is *visceral obesity.* Fat is deposited in vital or-gans like the heart, liver and kidneys. Women notice it as a "thickening" of their waistlines and find it very distressing. It commonly occurs in overweight women and makes it more difficult to lose weight. It can even occur in normal weight women who suddenly see their body shape changing from the "pear shape" of a younger woman to an "apple shape." This excess abdominal fat releases harmful leptin and ***tumor necro-sis factor alpha*** (TNF-alpha,) that oppose the action of insulin leading to a condition called insulin resistance that further increases the risk of heart disease. Insulin resistance can also lead to an increased incidence of diabetes mellitus which also increases heart disease.

Most people mistakenly think that heart attacks and strokes occur because the arteries get blocked with calcified plaque buildup. On the contrary, 80% of all heart attacks and isch-emic strokes are caused by blockage of an artery going to the heart or brain due to rupture of an unstable soft plaque. Visualize a soft plaque as a pimple on the inside lining of an artery. Because it's not calcified, the surface is soft and mushy like a pimple. Sudden rupture of the plaque releases inflam-matory substances inducing spasm/constriction of the artery and causing the blockage that results in a heart attack.

The best way to screen for risk of heart disease or stroke is with an ultrasound test called ***Carotid intima media thickness test*** (CIMT.) CIMT test is a valid and reliable screening test recommended by the *American Heart Association* and the *American College of Cardiology.* CIMT, a painless, noninvasive, fairly inexpensive tool, utilizes ultrasound to measure the thickness of the intima and media layers of the carotid arteries. These measurements are compared to a reference group of women your age to determine how rapidly your arteries are aging. If your arteries are aging prematurely, it provides an early warning that more aggressive measures need to be taken. CIMT is also able to detect the presence of soft plaque, the most dangerous form of plaque that can lead to heart attacks.

Women suffering severe or prolonged hot flashes have a higher risk of heart disease. This phenomenon occurs more commonly in women who experience an abrupt fall in estrogen as in surgical menopause. In a study following two groups of women who were or were not exhibiting severe flashes, the hot flash group had worsening progression in their CIMT values.

The good news is that when aggressive preventive measures are instituted, abnormalities can often be improved! Better to find out you have heart disease when it is a silent disease than when you are in the emergency room having a heart attack! This is why I monitor CIMTs in all my patients on a yearly basis to assess their progress. Importantly, understanding their abnormal CIMT motivates the patient to be more compliant with their program of medication, exercise, and healthy eating, especially when they see the abnormal CIMT improving.

The *Kronos Early Estrogen Prevention Study* (KEEPS) is underway to compare two regimens of HRT in 729 postmenopausal women who are within three years of menopause. It is a

randomized, placebo controlled, double-blinded trial following women for four years and will be completed in July 2012.
Participants will be randomized into one of three groups,
placebo, oral estrogen or topical estrogen with the latter two
combined with 200 mg of oral, cyclic, progesterone the first
12 days of each calendar month. The two estrogen groups will
receive either oral conjugated equine estrogens (Premarin)
0.45 mg or a topical estradiol 0.05 mg weekly patch (Climara).
All women will undergo CIMT testing and coronary calcium
scores to assess progression of heart disease. This study should
give us further valuable evidence of which HRT regimen offers
the most protection against heart disease.

Key Cardiovascular Changes Resulting From Estrogen Loss at Menopause

1. Worsening of Cholesterol: fall in beneficial HDL and rise
   in harmful LDL
2. Increased Fibrinogen and clumping of platelets leading to
   excess clot formation
3. Overgrowth of cells in blood vessel walls leading to
   plaque formation
4. Increase in chronic inflammation in blood vessels
5. Increase in blood pressure leading to hypertension
6. Increase in insulin resistance which accelerates heart disease & diabetes
7. Increased visceral fat causing "thickening" around the
   waistline and weight gain

Alzheimer's Disease, Poor Memory, and Mental Focus

Another symptom of estrogen deficiency many women fear
is the decline in memory and mental concentration. Our
mothers and grandmothers often accepted this as a necessary
consequence of aging. Postmenopausal women often describe

it as "brain fog" and "fuzzy thinking." They especially notice problems with word retrieval and remembering names and phone numbers they could easily recall before menopause.

When I'm on plane trips and women learn I'm a physician specializing in menopause, they usually tell me their stories. Earlier this year, I sat next to Jane, a PhD researcher, who works for a prominent east coast research institution. She had been menopausal for 3 years and was terrified of taking hormones because she was fearful of breast cancer. Jane lamented, *"Dr Johnson, I can't remember articles I've just read. I have to read and re-read them to make any sense of them. I keep incessant lists of everything to keep me on task. I'm afraid I'm going to lose my job!"* I reassured her about the risk-benefit ratio for estrogen, told her about topical HRT and advised her to follow-up with a menopause specialist.

On another plane trip this month, I sat next to Jackie, a woman in her 60s who told me about her experience when she became menopausal 10 years ago. Jackie said, *"I was having awful hot flashes and could not think straight. I became paranoid and frightened, and I was afraid to be in any social situations. I asked my young doctor for help but he just told me that was something normal that would eventually pass. I relied on advice from an older woman friend, long menopausal. I coped by refusing to go out of my house for six months and staying in bed most of the that time. My husband was worried sick about me until finally I felt a little better."*

I submit to you in the 21st century, this is not an acceptable way to treat fifty percent of our population who will all eventually go through this life stage. In addition to the suffering of these women, think of the lost productivity. When you don't have your mind, your quality of life is severely compromised.

When estrogen deficiency continues long-term, there is an increased risk for the development of Alzheimer's disease. In June 2008, the *Centers for Disease Control and Prevention* reported that AD is now the sixth leading cause of death in the United States, surpassing diabetes. There are currently five million Americans with AD or dementia and more than half of them are women. This total figure is expected to increase to 10 million as the Baby Boomers age.

Estrogen has the following effects on the brain:

1. Modulation of synapses, the special junctions where nerve cells communicate with each other
2. Increase of cerebral blood flow
3. Mediation of important neurotransmitters and hormones
4. Protection against apoptosis (programmed cell death)
5. Increase in anti-inflammatory actions
6. Antioxidant effects

There are estradiol receptors throughout the brain especially in the basal forebrain located near the bottom of the front of the brain. This area includes the *hippocampus* that is important for memory and learning.

There is clearly an association between the length of time a woman maintains her own estrogen production and her ability to have normal mental focus and memory. When women undergo surgical menopause at an early age and do not take estrogen, they have a sharper decline in these mental functions than women who undergo natural menopause. A *Mayo Clinic* study of 3000 women followed for 30 years found that women who had one or both ovaries removed before menopause and did not take estrogen were more likely to develop dementia and Parkinson's Disease.

Despite the biologic importance of estradiol in a woman's mental function, studies in women receiving HRT have been less conclusive. The Nurses' Health Study of 13,087 postmenopausal women followed for eight years showed no appreciable mental benefits in women who took oral estrogen or estrogen/synthetic progestin as compared to those on no HRT. On the contrary, they showed an actual increased risk of mental decline in those women who started HRT at an older age.
A possible mechanism for this is that oral estrogen increases C-reactive protein that has been associated with increased dementia. A few smaller studies have shown a modest benefit in improving cognitive function. The *WHI Memory Study* showed worsening of dementia in women taking Prempro; however, the dementia appears to be related to the use of continuous combined estrogen plus *medroxyprogesterone acetate* (MPA). MPA has been found to reduce mental performance in both animal and human studies. See previous chapter on *Risks of Adding Oral Synthetic Progestins*.

A *positron emission tomography* (PET) scan is a diagnostic imaging scan that uses low-dose radioactive sugar to measure functional brain activity. PET scans can be used to demonstrate patterns associated with *Alzheimer's disease* (AD). In a randomized study of 81 younger post menopausal women at risk for Alzheimer's disease all were started on estrogen at the beginning of the study. A baseline PET scan was done and then half the group was randomized to continue on estrogen for two years while the other group had estrogen discontinued. Metabolic activity in brain regions most altered in AD was largely preserved in the women who continued estrogen but declined in those who stopped estrogen. In the women who continued estrogen brain activity in the frontal cortex actually increased.

To achieve the optimal brain protective effect of estrogen, women are advised to start on topical estrogen soon after menopause. In light of the lack of protection seen in the *WHI Memory Study*, it seems prudent to initiate topical estradiol. In women with an intact uterus, cyclic progesterone should be used over a synthetic progestin. Women who start estrogen after age 60 have no reduction in their risk of AD probably because they have already developed degenerative brain loss.

The Cache County Study on Memory, Health and Aging has been following a group of 5,092 seniors in rural, northeastern Utah since 1995 to determine the development of Alzheimer's disease. In 2005 they published findings showing an increased risk of developing AD when you carry a gene called *Apolipoprotein E* (ApoE4.) If you inherit an ApoE4 gene from each parent, your gene type is called ApoE 4/4. If you only receive one ApoE4, your type is ApoE 3/4 or ApoE 2/4.

The *Cache study* also reported medications that may reduce the risk of developing Alzheimer's disease. Use of aspirin and *non-steroidal anti-inflammatory agents* (NSAIDS) like ibuprofen were associated with a reduced prevalence of AD by about 50%. Use of Vitamin E and vitamin C showed a decreased prevalence of AD but only if they were both used in combination. Estrogen use reduced AD risk by 50%, and in women without dementia, estrogen use improved cognitive performance.

While estrogen has been shown to *prevent* the occurrence of Alzheimer's disease, in studies specifically evaluating the effect of oral estrogen in women with established AD, no effect on progression of the disease was seen. A few small studies have shown topical estrogen positively influences postmenopausal memory and may offer some protective effect against the mental decline seen in AD.

We have seen differences between oral and topical estrogen, and between progesterone and synthetic progestins, in the risks of breast cancer and heart disease. It is tempting to speculate that this may also explain the lack of clear benefit of oral estrogen in reducing the risk of mental decline and Alzheimer's disease. Future research on treatment for AD should focus on such variables as the route of estrogen administration, the form of estrogen (conjugated estrogens versus estradiol), when estrogen is initiated following menopause, duration of estrogen treatment, and the effects of opposed versus unopposed estrogen to define which HRT regimens may have a benefit.

Osteoporosis

After menopause without the use of estrogen, a woman can lose up to 20% of her bone mass. This increases her risk for osteoporosis leading to loss of height, hip fractures, chronic pain, and disability. Of women who suffer hip fractures, 24 percent die of complications within a year of the injury. Osteoporosis of the spine leads to the familiar *"dowager's hump."* A dowager's hump is a prominence on the back resulting from collapse of the spine from spontaneous vertebral fractures. When it's severe, the woman is totally bent over and cannot stand up straight. It is tragic to see a woman suffering from something that could have been prevented.

A recent British study estimated the lifetime risk for any fracture to be 53.2% at age 50 among women not taking estrogen. In comparison, the estimated lifetime risk for endometrial carcinoma for a 50-year-old woman is 2.6%, for breast cancer 10%, for coronary artery disease 46%, and for stroke 20%.

Prevention of osteoporosis was the first FDA-approved indication for estrogen therapy. In the *Million Women Study*, a prospective, cohort study of over one million women, all taking different formulations of estrogen, including oral and transdermal, were associated with a lower risk of hip and vertebral fractures. While not FDA-approved for this indication, estrogen is also effective for treatment of osteoporosis. In a study of 75 women treated with either topical estradiol or placebo for one year, the estrogen group had an increased bone density in hip and spine and 50% fewer fractures.

Estrogen is even effective at protecting bones when started after age 75. One study in 67 elderly women over 75 years old treated with estrogen for nine months showed improvement in bone density in the hip and spine compared to placebo. Improvements in bone density are seen even with ultra low doses of estrogen, like 0.25 mg of oral estradiol or a 0.014 mg estradiol patch. At such low doses there appears to be no stimulation to the uterine lining.

How does estrogen work to prevent osteoporosis? When people think of bones, they may have a visual image of the skeleton that you studied in biology class. They see the skeleton as inanimate, solid scaffolding that simply holds up the rest of the body. Nothing could be further from the truth. Bones are active living tissues maintained by a continuous balance between two types of bone cells, *osteoclasts* and *osteoblasts* that work upon an internal collagen framework. Osteoclasts break down bone (resorption) while osteoblasts build bone onto the collagen framework. When bones are injured, osteoclasts rush in to remove the damaged bone and osteoblasts deposit new bone to repair it.

Most women are very familiar with *collagen* because it is an important support structure which plumps up the skin preventing wrinkles. However, few are aware that collagen is also present in fingernails, hair, tendons and importantly, in bone. Since collagen normally declines with aging, reduction in the collagen framework can further weaken the bone leading to "brittle bones" commonly seen in elderly individuals. In animal studies, loss of estrogen increases immune cells that produce a protein called *tumor necrosis factor* (TNF) that increases the formation of osteoclasts. With an increase in osteoclasts over osteoblasts, the net result is bone resorption or bone loss leading to osteoporosis. Estrogen decreases this accelerated bone resorption and also plays a role in improving calcium absorption in the intestine.

Lifestyle measures which will further increase bone density include weight-bearing exercise, taking in adequate dietary calcium, taking adequate vitamin D, and treating inflammatory conditions that cause increased bone loss.

Diabetes

According to the *American Diabetes Association*, diabetes was the sixth leading cause of death in 2007. Ninety-five percent of diabetes is type-2 that develops in older people or at any age in overweight people. Diabetes dramatically increases the risk for heart disease and stroke.

Women who do not take HRT have up to a 30% increased risk of developing type-2 diabetes. Use of estrogen or estrogen plus a progestin/progesterone is associated with a decrease in the risk for type-2 diabetes.

Women in their forties or fifties often complain about a tendency to gain weight, especially when they don't take hormones. I recall Greta, a 38 year-old menopausal woman with obesity, diabetes, high blood pressure, and sleep apnea. She was only five feet tall and weighed 200 pounds. She told me, *"When I was growing up I was skinny and barely weighted 100 pounds soaking wet! I could eat as much as the football players and never gained a pound. In my late 20s, I started having heavy bleeding from fibroids and when I was 28 years old, everything was taken out. No one ever told me I needed estrogen. Within a year of my hysterectomy, I gained 100 pounds and developed severe depression. My husband left me soon after that. A doctor finally gave me oral estrogen when I was 32 and I felt better but couldn't lose the weight. I was diagnosed with diabetes and high blood pressure when I was 35."* Changing Greta to topical HRT and correcting her sleep apnea started her recovery toward losing weight and improving control of her blood pressure and diabetes. However, it saddens me that she suffered needlessly for ten years before getting help.

Weight gain with a change in body composition favoring central or visceral obesity accompanies menopause. Women lament the fact they start having thickening around their midriff! With loss of estrogen comes an increase in fasting glucose and the development of insulin resistance leading to diabetes in genetically susceptible women. *Insulin resistance* is a condition where the body becomes "desensitized" to the actions of insulin. Because insulin is a vital hormone, the pancreas responds by making more insulin. This satisfies the need for insulin action but at the expense of higher circulating levels of insulin. High levels of insulin signal fat cells to conserve fat stores and to convert new food into more fat! This is not a signal you want going to your fat cells!

In individuals who are genetically predisposed to diabetes, this relentless drive for more and more insulin production eventually exhausts the pancreas leading to the onset of diabetes. Even if they never develop diabetes, the presence of ongoing insulin resistance is associated with continued weight gain and accelerates the risk of heart disease, cancer and strokes.

In a group of 505 normal weight non-diabetic women, menopause was the determining factor and not age that was associated with insulin resistance. *Leptin*, a hormone made in fat cells is responsible for regulating appetite and metabolism. Although leptin is a hormone that reduces appetite, obese people tend to have elevated leptin levels and also seem to develop resistance to the effects of leptin.

A prospective study of 44 healthy postmenopausal women randomized to receive either no treatment or topical estradiol 0.05 mg per day combined with a cyclic progestin were followed for one year. Untreated postmenopausal women had an increase in total and percent body fat and increased visceral body fat. Untreated postmenopausal women also showed corresponding increases in serum leptin levels. The women receiving topical estradiol had no increase in leptin and had no increase in body fat.

Colon Cancer

The use of HRT reduces the incidence of and mortality from colon cancer by about 30 to 50%. This benefit was also seen in the WHI study, which showed a 50% reduction in risk after three years in the combined estrogen/progestin group but not in the estrogen only group. However, the WHI women receiving Prempro diagnosed with colon cancer during the study tended to exhibit a higher percentage of local and metastatic spread of their cancer. The Nurses Health Study of 59,002 postmenopausal women followed for 14 years showed a 35% decreased incidence of colon cancer with combined estrogen/ progestin. Because estrogen offers protection against colon cancer, this perhaps explains why giving anti-estrogen drugs like *tamoxifen* increases the incidence of colorectal cancer by 15 to 40%.

Reduced Pulmonary Function

Studies show that menopausal women who do not take estrogen experience a loss of lung alveoli, the air sacs in the lungs where oxygen is absorbed into the blood. This affects their breathing efficiency and oxygen exchange. This probably explains why post menopausal women off hormones sometimes notice they are more prone to bronchial infections, shortness of breath and may even experience a decline in their singing voices. Elegant studies by Dr. Donald Massaro of Georgetown Medical School show the alveoli actually grow back after the estrogen is resumed which explains the improvement in symptoms.

Giving estrogen plus progesterone or estrogen alone to post-menopausal women improves measurements of lung function, including forced vital capacity and *forced expiratory volume* (FEV1). FEV1 is a test that measures the volume of air that a person can exhale in one second of forced expiration. Low ovarian hormones are associated with an increased incidence of *chronic obstructive pulmonary disease* (COPD) due to loss of alveoli.

While HRT improves pulmonary function, some studies show that HRT can be associated with new onset asthma and worsening of FEV1. I have not personally seen this in my patients on topical estradiol, but it is reported in the literature with oral contraceptives and all forms of hormone replacement therapy.

Osteoarthritis

Loss of estrogen leads to deterioration of joint cartilage leading to joint stiffness, pain, and decreased quality of life. Estrogen alone offers protection against osteoarthritis and the need for joint replacements. When progestin is added to estrogen this protection is reduced. A study of 4000 women on HRT for longer than ten years showed a 40% lower risk of osteoarthritis of the hip compared to women on no HRT. Another study showed similar protection from osteoarthritis of the knee.

Falls

Women over the age of 50 have an increased incidence of wrist fractures resulting from falls. Lack of estrogen contributes to problems with balance, resulting in more falls. In one study of 1523 women on no HRT, it was noted that those women having more significant hot flashes had more problems with balance. One study showed an improvement in balance in women on topical estradiol compared to those on no HRT. Another study using oral Premarin showed no improvement in balance compared to no HRT.

Gout

In the Nurses' Health Study, a prospective study of 92,535 women followed for 16 years, 1603 new cases of gout were diagnosed during the study period. Since gout can also be affected by such risk factors as age, body mass index, diuretic use, hypertension, alcohol intake, and dietary intake, these factors were also taken into consideration in comparing the different groups. Women under age 45 had an incidence of gout of 0.6 per 1000 compared to 2.5 in women over 75 years of age. Women who experienced menopause under the age of 45 had an increased relative risk of 1.62 compared to those who became menopausal at ages 50 to 54 who had a relative risk for gout of 1.0. While HRT was not analyzed by type, menopausal women receiving any HRT had a reduced relative risk of 0.82 for developing gout.

Increased Mortality

Observational studies have generally reported an overall reduction in mortality from HRT primarily as a result of lessening heart disease. However, some of this decrease in mortality has been attributed to the fact that women taking HRT (having consulted a physician for treatment) are more likely to be conscientious about their health and thus have healthier lifestyles regarding diet and exercise and better compliance with physician office visits and medications. A *meta-analysis* of 30 randomized, controlled trials comparing women receiving HRT to those on no HRT showed a 40% reduced mortality in women who started HRT at less than 60 years of age or were within 10 years of menopause onset. No improvement in mortality was seen in those studies where the women first started HRT at an average age greater than 60.

If you are to take HRT,
which one to choose

Chapter 23

Why a bioidentical product?

If after reviewing the risks and benefits of estrogen, you have decided you want to take HRT, let me tell you why I recommend bioidentical HRT. It is a therapy I have utilized in the 100,000 female patient visits that I have managed over the past 25 years since **pharmaceutical topical estradiol** was first introduced in 1986. I have had ample opportunity to see what therapies achieve results and what women tolerate with the fewest side effects.

An important concept regarding hormone therapy is that unlike most other prescription medicines, hormones are part of our biological make-up and are essential to the intrinsic function of our bodies. We've learned in previous chapters of the myriad biological actions of estradiol, progesterone and testosterone in a woman's body. We have also seen that many of these actions are mediated through downstream byproducts of estradiol. So doesn't it make more sense to restore what's deficient rather than cluttering this complex, intricate system with an imitation, "wannabe" hormone?

Female hormones have been in our bodies since we went through puberty. It is part of our original design since the beginning of time. Yes, there are some safety concerns about estrogen. So logically, if you've made the decision to take HRT, it makes sense to choose what appears to be the safer option. I have tried to fairly represent that bioidentical HRT is not without risks but the risks appear to be less with topical estradiol and progesterone than with imitation HRT. Should we wait another 20 years until large definitive, double-blind, placebo-controlled randomized studies produce more data in support of these findings? While some of the data are not supported by such scientifically rigorous studies, as a prudent physician needing to care for my patients today, I feel compelled to act on what is currently known and act accordingly, making adjustments as additional new studies provide us with more information.

To those naysayers who contend that pregnant horse urine is "natural," I choose the very same hormones, estradiol, proges- terone, and testosterone that are present in a human woman's body, not hormones from animals. Furthermore, you can take any natural substance that exists in the body, give it in excess amounts, and cause disease or death. For instance, something as essential to life as oxygen and water, given in excess, can be fatal. It is all about balance and respecting the normal physiol- ogy of the body. That is the goal of endocrinology, a specialty that deals with diagnosing and treating diseases caused by too much or too little hormone(s.)

Women are often surprised to learn that the bioidentical hormones, estradiol and progesterone, are available from pharmaceutical companies. That's because the term "bioi- dentical hormone replacement" is often given a negative connotation. It often becomes a clash between pharmaceu- tical companies and compounding pharmacists.

Most pharmacists dispense prescription medications that are manufactured by pharmaceutical companies. Compounding pharmacists are trained to make individual hormone products from bulk raw materials. The physician writes a prescription for a particular hormone preparation and the pharmacist mixes it to those specifications. Pharmaceutical companies correctly assert that they have to meet higher manufacturing standards for quality control than compounding pharmacists. Pharmaceutical companies complain compounded hormone products are often given to women without the attendant information that outlines risks.

I have no bias against pharmaceutical companies. They provide us with lifesaving and innovative therapies. However, I won't prescribe the most commonly prescribed HRT - Prempro or any oral estrogen - because it is not as effective as topical therapy and is associated with more side effects. As an advocate for my patients, it is my ethical responsibility to prescribe the safer, more effective therapy, and that principle governs all my professional decisions. The appropriateness of my choices has been demonstrated in the medical literature, and I have personally observed it in the thousands of patients I have treated over my clinical career.

Having been a pharmacist, I am very supportive of the important role of compounding pharmacists. However, if I have a choice of a compounded or pharmaceutical bioidentical hormone product, I will always choose the pharmaceutical product because they have to meet stricter standards of quality control, and I achieve more consistent results when I monitor blood levels.

Compounding pharmacists play an important role in providing products for patients with allergies and other special needs. They can also compound products that are not commercially available. Pharmaceutical companies sometimes withdraw drugs from the market not because of poor efficacy but because there may not be enough market demand for their product. **If a physician chooses to prescribe compounded hormones, it is imperative that blood levels be monitored**. These patients need to be monitored in the same manner as any other patient receiving HRT. Patients also need to be informed that compounded HRT carries the same risks as pharmaceutical bioidentical hormones.

Talking to Your Doctor

Informing yourself of the risks and benefits of bioidentical HRT is important but since these are all prescription medicines, you will ultimately require the cooperation and advice of your physician. Your own physician can advise you if you have particular health issues which constitute a relative contraindication to bioidentical HRT. If you are having many menopausal symptoms, he/she will be more likely to prescribe HRT. All physicians want the best for their patients and are usually willing to "listen to" and consider reasonable requests. If your physician believes that hormones are in your best interest, pharmaceutical bioidentical HRT is a good choice. Make a list of all your questions ahead of time and tell the scheduling person that you want an appointment to discuss hormone therapy. If you found this book helpful, take a copy to your physician. Do not hesitate to seek out additional medical opinions about your individual condition - caring physicians will assist you in doing so.

This book can increase your awareness of how hormones contribute to optimal health. **Healing starts with your belief that it is possible.** Use this book as a guide to educate yourself about your treatment options so you can ask meaningful questions and become a better partner in working with your physician.

FAQs ABOUT BIOIDENTICAL HRT

Q. What if I'm on Prempro and want to change to bioidentical hormones. Can I still get benefit?

Patients see me who have been on Prempro for years and are not feeling well. They are anxious to know if changing to bioidentical HRT will enable them to regain their good health. Prempro and other forms of combined HRT have been associated with increased side effects, primarily because of the daily dose of progestin and also from the use of oral estrogen. According to a 2009 study, the increased risk of breast cancer dropped to baseline within two years of stopping Prempro. Changing to bioidentical HRT will usually cause a woman to feel better and often improves various parameters including blood pressure, cholesterol, weight gain, sleep, and other measures.

Obviously, the sooner she changes to a safer program, the better. I must reiterate however, that bioidentical HRT is not without risk. That's why it is a prescription medication and should be carefully considered and monitored by your physician.

Q. I never took hormones after menopause. Is it too late for me?

At the time of menopause, each woman has a window of opportunity during which she needs to make the important decision of whether to take hormones. As the estrogen levels fall, her body begins to go through degenerative changes that accelerate her risk of heart disease along with the other changes we have previously described. The sooner a woman starts HRT after menopause, the fewer degenerative changes she will experience. If a woman waits 10 years to start HRT, the heart protection from estrogen is greatly diminished. The same applies to brain protection; once brain cells have been lost, it becomes difficult to retrieve normal function. However, for protecting bones, estrogen is effective even when started after age 75.

However, I would like to stress that each woman is an individual and if there are no contraindications to trying hormones, consider trying topical estradiol for a year to see if you experience any improvements. I recall Cora, an 82 year-old woman who was brought to me by her daughter June. Cora had never taken hormones after menopause.

June said, *"Mom has always been so vibrant, energetic and happy and she loved to do gardening. However, for the past six months she just sits in a rocker and stares at the wall. I've taken her to several doctors and they have all told me that everything's normal but this is not normal for my mother! Is there anything you can do to help her?"* I examined her mother and the only abnormal lab result was her lack of estrogen. I told June, *"I'm not sure how much benefit we can expect to see but let's try her on estrogen and see how she responds".* A mere three months later, now with therapeutic estrogen levels, June told me with excitement, *"I have my mother back! She's smiling and happy and back to her old self."* Cora taught me to never give up on a patient just because they are older. Everyone deserves a chance to be better. People deserve to be treated as individuals not as statistics on a bell-shaped curve. I challenge my patients to become the outliers who defy the odds and do better than expected.

Q. How long can I safely stay on my hormone therapy?

I am frequently asked this question, and I usually ask the woman, *"How long do you want to continue to feel well?"* In all seriousness, there are no long-term studies that enable me to answer this question. Taking hormones less than five years seems to carry very little risk. However, the longer you take hormones the higher your risk.

The *North American Menopause Society* and the *Endocrine Society* have addressed this issue. They recommend that all women be informed of potential risks and benefits and given the lowest effective dose consistent with treatment goals. If a woman wishes to continue HRT for an extended period of time, this is acceptable if she and her physician believe that the benefits of continuing HRT outweigh the risks. A woman's decision to initiate or continue HRT must be based on her own unique circumstances and risks. Many of the available studies have not attempted to evaluate the differences in risks among the different HRT regiments. However, new studies are beginning to appear that help sort out the risks for the different types of HRT. In a sense, the Baby Boomers are the "test generation" that started HRT in larger numbers. We will be the first to see the consequences, positive and negative, of being on HRT for 20, 30, and 40 years.

Q. Why didn't my Ob-Gyn start me on this program?

When I see a woman who is doing poorly on Prempro or oral estrogen and she improves after changing to topical HRT, she is often angry with her previous doctor. Patients sometimes have naive expectations that one doctor should know everything. While some gynecologists specialize in menopause, most Ob-Gyns in private practice are generalists and care for a wide range of women's health problems. Furthermore, Ob-Gyns are first and foremost surgeons and in their residency training must acquire the skills to perform gynecological surgery and deliver babies, neither of which I can do. It's unfair to expect that in addition to keeping up with the literature in obstetrics and surgical gynecology, an Ob-Gyn should also keep up with all the literature in endocrinology and internal medicine.

My training in internal medicine and endocrinology gives me expertise in the medical management of chronic hormone problems. Because of my interest in menopause, I am especially mindful of keeping up with this literature. However, I greatly rely on gynecologists to help me with patients who require diagnostic procedures or surgery.

I could not properly manage my patients without their expertise. Once patients understand that no one physician can know everything, they have a better appreciation of their gynecologists and all the other physicians who may care for them.

Q. Do younger women who undergo premature or surgical menopause have the same risks as women who go through natural menopause?

The *North American Menopause Society* and the *Endocrine Society* have also addressed this issue as an area of concern. They caution that data from such large trials as WHI and HERS should not be extrapolated to younger postmenopausal woman who initiate HRT shortly after menopause. WHI involved older women with a mean age of 63 who were asymptomatic and had never taken HRT. The HERS study was a group of women with a mean age of 67 who all had known heart disease.They also recommend that such studies not be applied to women who experience premature menopause at ages younger than 40. Since women with early menopause will generally be on HRT for a longer period of time, it's even more important that they choose the safest form of therapy which at this time, appears to be topical bioidentical HRT.

Chapter 24

Why I Have Always Used Topical Estradiol

Topical delivery of hormones is accomplished through a patch, cream or gel applied to the skin. Many of the landmark studies on topical estradiol were done by Dr. Howard Judd and Dr. David Meldrum from UCLA. As a medical student, Dr. Meldrum was a mentor to me so I became aware of the adverse side effects of oral estrogen early in my career. When I began my private medical practice in 1986, topical estradiol was an obvious choice for my patients.

Topical therapy comes closer to mimicking the way estradiol is delivered by the ovaries. In a normal premenopausal woman, estradiol is never deposited in the stomach once a day. Rather, the ovaries release small amounts of estradiol directly into the bloodstream throughout the day. Topical patches and creams are the closest way we have of approximating this elegant, delivery system.

After any medicine is swallowed, it is absorbed into the digestive system and is metabolized in the liver before it reaches the rest of the body. This aspect of drug metabolism is called the *"first-pass effect"* and often markedly reduces the amount of active drug reaching the rest of the body. For example, an oral dose of one mg of oral estradiol must be given to achieve the same therapeutic blood levels as one-tenth mg of topical estradiol. After an oral dose of one mg of micronized estradiol, blood estradiol levels peak at four to five hours and by eight to 10 hours return to baseline. This often results in recurrence of low estrogen symptoms. Estrogen patches or creams produce more consistent, steady state blood levels.

Furthermore, adverse side effects occur from exposing the liver to abnormally high levels of estrogen. For more discussion on the *Risks from Oral Estrogen* go to Chapter 20.

PROBLEMS SOMETIMES ENCOUNTERED WITH ESTROGEN

Estrogen Excess

Estrogen excess with inappropriately high estradiol levels can be caused by HRT that is improperly prescribed or delivered. I've seen such symptoms more frequently in women after they've received estrogen injections or pellets.

For estradiol pellets, a small incision is made in the woman's buttock and several estrogen pellets are implanted which release estradiol over one to three months. I have never utilized this type of HRT, but some practitioners report good results with this type of therapy. However, in my personal experience with these patients, they exhibited enormously high levels of estrogen in the range of 2000 pg/ml (normal is 50-70). Understandably, these women sought me out because they were not doing well with estrogen pellets so perhaps others do well. In four of the women, it took them each over two years from the last estrogen pellet implant before their estradiol levels dropped to physiologic range. Apparently, these women had impaired ability to metabolize the estrogen pellets that resulted in excessive estrogen accumulation. Because high estrogen levels have been associated with a higher risk of breast and uterine cancer, estrogen excess should be avoided.

Signs and Symptoms of Excess Estrogen

1. Breast Tenderness & Swelling
2. Nausea or Vomiting
3. Weight Gain
4. Fluid Retention or swelling
5. Sense of Heaviness
6. Pounding Headaches
7. Paradoxical Hot Flashes, Sweats, Insomnia
8. Anxiety or Depression
9. Mood swings and irritability
10. Palpitations
11. Excess Vaginal Bleeding
12. Recurrent Vaginal Yeast Infections
13. Bloating

At very high estrogen levels, an interesting phenomenon occurs in that the woman may have a paradoxical **increase** in
hot flashes, insomnia and other symptoms more typically
seen with a low estrogen state. When the body is exposed
to enormously high hormone levels, the body has a protective mechanism that shuts off the estrogen receptors and this
effect is often referred to as a *"down regulation of estrogen
receptors."* This may explain why these women often exhibit
hot flashes and insomnia despite high estrogen levels. This is
another reason to monitor blood estradiol levels and aim for
an optimal dose that is neither too high or too low.

Hyperprolactinemia

Despite appropriate estradiol levels, symptoms similar to those
of estrogen excess can also occur in women with elevations
in *prolactin*, a pituitary hormone, which increases a woman's
sensitivity to normal doses of estrogen. If prolactin is significantly elevated, these women require a diagnostic evaluation to

exclude a prolactin-secreting pituitary tumor. Various medications, trauma to the chest and even stress can result in modest elevations in prolactin levels and should be evaluated by your endocrinologist and treated accordingly. After correcting hyperprolactinemia, a woman can generally tolerate typical doses of estradiol replacement therapy.

PHARMACEUTICAL ESTRADIOL PREPARATIONS

Topical Estradiol Patches

Patches are usually my first choice because of their convenience. I generally prefer the twice-weekly patches because of less skin irritation. I typically have the woman change her patch every Sunday night and Thursday morning. The twice-weekly patches include *Alora, Esclim, Estraderm* and *Vivelle Dot. Climara* and *Menostar* are changed once a week. *Menostar* is a ultra low dose estradiol patch releasing 0.014 mg/day.

If you love long, hot soaks in a jacuzzi or bath, patches may not be a good choice. Hot water leaches estrogen from the patch. I've documented sub-therapeutic estradiol levels in such cases. When the women changed to showers, estradiol levels became therapeutic. If a woman misses her baths but wants to use patches, a good compromise is to take baths on Sundays and Wednesdays (just before she's ready for a new patch) and take showers the other days. Vigorous exercise with lots of sweating or very hot summer temperatures may require an upward adjustment in your dosage. Since we have such hot summers in Dallas, I have some very physically active women who require a stronger dose patch in the summer. Women who develop local skin reactions from the patch will sometimes tolerate a different brand of patch. If they do not tolerate any patch, they should be changed to an estradiol gel or cream.

TIPS ON WEARING THE ESTRADIOL PATCH

1. Make sure the skin is clean and dry with no rashes or cuts at the application site.
2. Adherence is improved by gently treating the area with alcohol prior to application of the patch and letting the skin dry. This is especially important if you apply body lotion, powders or oils to your skin.
3. The patch should be applied below the waist to the abdomen or buttock. Don't put the patch near a panty line or at the waist line. Never apply the patch to the breasts.
4. Pull away half the backing and apply the patch to your skin without touching the adhesive side. Remove the other half of the backing and pat down the patch.
5. Gently apply rubbing motions to the patch to ensure that the patch has adhered well to the skin.
6. Don't apply lotions or oils near the patch because it may be likely to fall off.
7. You can swim or shower without disrupting the patch. Baths are not advisable because the hot water leaches estrogen from the patch.
8. Rotate sides so that the patch is not applied to the same site.
9. If you get redness, itching or hives at the site of the patch, don't resort to chronic use of cortisone cream. It's better to try a different brand of patch or change to a gel or cream.

Estradiol Topical Gels and Creams

Women who do not tolerate patches should change to gels or creams. There are a variety of pharmaceutical estradiol preparations with varying amounts of estradiol and the different gels and creams may have different efficiencies of absorption. This can be problematic when you are switching from one product to another. For example, one pump of *Estragel*, an alcohol-based gel contains 0.75 mg of estradiol per dose and delivers 0.035 mg of estradiol. Compare that to *Estrasorb*, a soy-based emulsion in a packet containing 4.35 mg of estradiol which delivers only 0.025 mg of estradiol. It's best to go by the amount of estradiol delivered and the resulting blood levels. Each product has its own unique features that some women may prefer over others. All of these products are generally dosed once daily. The pharmaceutical estradiol products which come as a cream are: *Divigel*, *Estrasorb*, and *Elestrin*. *Estragel* is available as a gel formulation and *Evamist* is a topical spray product.

However, keep in mind the variance in absorption from one product to another. Thin active women generally require higher doses than obese women. The creams and gels are applied to the skin but never to the breasts. Most women apply them to the buttocks, thighs or forearms.

COMPOUNDED ORAL AND TOPICAL ESTRADIOL

I have already explained in prior sections why I prefer topical over oral estradiol. While I prefer pharmaceutical topical estradiol because of its consistency and quality control, compounded estradiol creams and gels could be safely used *provided blood estradiol levels are being monitored*. However, such monitoring is currently not a common practice because I frequently see women on compounded estradiol products (from other physicians) with an estradiol level of zero! Because compounded estradiol products are generic they are much less costly than brand-name pharmaceutical estradiol. This may be an important consideration for some women.

OTHER ESTRADIOL PRODUCTS

Vaginal Preparations

Vaginal estradiol preparations are useful for women with symptoms including vaginal dryness, painful intercourse, recurrent urinary tract infections, stress or urge incontinence, and urinary frequency or urgency. These products are indicated when vaginal or bladder symptoms persist despite the woman's use of systemic HRT like topical or oral estrogen. They are generally dosed daily for two weeks and then a maintenance dose of two to three times weekly is sufficient. For women on systemic estradiol concerned about taking the minimal dose of estrogen, these preparations do provide another exposure to estradiol, the most potent form of estrogen.

Estradiol Vaginal cream

Estrace 0.1 mg estradiol per gram

Estradiol Vaginal Tablet

Vagifem 0.025 mg estradiol per tablet *(discontinued in July 2010)*

Vagifem 0.010 mg estradiol per tablet

Vaginal Ring

Estring - 0.0075 mg estradiol/day released over 3 months

Intravaginal ring

Femring - 0.05 mg estradiol/day over 3 months.

Femring - 0.1 mg estradiol/day over 3 months

(In women with an intact uterus these two products requires the addition of progesterone.)

Estradiol Injections

Estrogen injections can be given monthly for replacement. I do not utilize this therapy because it tends to produce very high estradiol levels after the injection and very low levels by the time the next injection is due. High estrogen levels have been associated with a higher risk of breast and uterine cancer.

Oral Estradiol Preparations

Oral estradiol is a bioidentical preparation, but I do not use any oral estrogen products in my practice because of the increased risks of oral compared to topical estradiol. Oral estrogen preparations have an increased conversion to estrone that is likely related to the higher doses required for oral estradiol. Since estrone is an active byproduct, we aim for the lowest estrogen level for a given effect. Hence, my preference for topical estradiol. There are many pharmaceutical topical estradiol preparations from which to choose. Since 1986 when pharmaceutical topical preparations were introduced, I have found it is rare to find a woman that cannot be managed with a topical preparation. Oral estradiol products include *Estrace, Gynodiol* and various generic estradiol preparations.

SYNTHETIC ESTROGEN OR ESTROGEN/PROGESTIN PREPARATIONS

None of the following preparations are bioidentical but I list them simply to help you identify the appropriate category into which each fits.

Oral Synthetic Estrogen Preparations

Oral synthetic estrogen products include **Premarin**, a mixture of conjugated equine estrogens made from the urine of pregnant horses.

Conjugated synthetic estrogens are made from plant sources and include *Cenestin* and *Enjuvia*.

Oral esterified estrogens are found in *Ogen, Estratab, Ortho-Est* and *Menest*.

Oral Synthetic Estrogens Combined with Oral Synthetic Progestins

Conjugated Equine Estrogens with Synthetic Progestins

The most commonly prescribed synthetic hormone in the US is *PremPro*, a combination of conjugated equine estrogens (estrogen from pregnant horses) and medroxyprogesterone. This is the preparation used in the Women's Health Initiative (WHI) study. Other estrogen/progestin combinations include *Prefest, Activella, FemHRT,* and *Angeliq*.

Oral estrogen-testosterone combinations:

Estratest, Estratest HS, Syntest DS, Syntest HS

Combination Estradiol/Progestin Patches

This group of patches combines topical estradiol with a topical synthetic progestin and they are mostly intended for continuous use. Because of the increased risks that have been reported with adding an oral daily progestin, I do not utilize patches that deliver daily progestin. While the risk of adding a topical daily progestin may only be theoretical, I think it is prudent to select a cyclic progestin until there are studies demonstrating comparable safety with topical continuous progestin.

These combination patches include *Combi-Patch* and *Climara Pro*. It is important to know *Climara Pro* only comes in a strength intended for continuous use.

Combi-Patch is available in two strengths, one intended for continuous use, estradiol 0.05 mg with 0.125 mg of norethindrone. Another *Combi-Patch* preparation containing 0.05 mg of estradiol with 0.25 mg of norethindrone is available for cyclic use.

Topical Estradiol With Cyclic Progestin

Recall that when using estrogen in any woman with an intact uterus, progesterone is always given to protect against endometrial cancer. In the premenopausal woman, the body's natural way of protecting against endometrial cancer is by the cleansing of the uterus with the monthly period. The monthly menstrual flow is the discharge of the excess build-of the uterine lining.

We mimic this natural protective process by adding either oral or vaginal progesterone to the estrogen for the first two weeks of each calendar month. A small predictable, menstrual period occurs each month within one to two days after the progesterone has been stopped. When an appropriate menstrual period does not occur following cyclic oral or vaginal progesterone, a combination patch called *Combi-Patch* 0.05 mg of estradiol and 0.25 mg of norethindrone can be used for cyclic therapy. If the woman is on a twice weekly patch of estradiol, she changes to *Combi-Patch* 0.05/0.25 mg twice weekly for the first four patches of each calendar month. To use this method you must use the *Combi-Patch* 0.05mg/0.25 mg which is the only combination patch intended for cyclic use. A predictable menstrual period will occur within two days after removing the fourth patch and changing back to the estradiol patch.

This method works best when the woman is on an estradiol 0.05 mg patch. If she is taking less than a 0.05 mg patch, this protocol is not advisable because she will be exceeding the estradiol dosage during those 14 days. If her estradiol dosage is greater than 0.05 mg, this is easily remedied by having her cut her estradiol patch and applying an extra patch with the *Combi-Patch* to equal the estradiol dose she typically takes. For example, if the woman requires a 0.1 mg estradiol patch, when changing to the *Combi-Patch*, cut the 0.1 mg estradiol patch in half lengthwise and apply that 1/2 patch along with each *Combi-Patch*.

Topical Birth Control Patch

When the topical *Ortha-Evra* was first released, I was hopeful that it would have the same advantage of avoiding the "first pass effect" on the liver much like topical estradiol. However, recent studies show that the adverse changes on vascular risk markers are the same in women who use *Ortha-Evra* and a comparable dose of the oral combined hormones. This occurs because the estrogen in *Ortho-Evra* is ethinyl estradiol, a more potent synthetic estrogen with a long duration of action that causes adverse effects to the liver.

Chapter 25

Progesterone - A necessary addition
if you have a uterus

A History Lesson

When the first estrogen (Premarin) was introduced in 1942, a woman with an intact uterus was treated with estrogen only without the use of progesterone. This practice is called "unopposed estrogen." After about 10 years of giving unopposed estrogen to millions of women, it became apparent that women were experiencing a high rate of uterine cancer. Studies showed this was caused by the lack of progesterone, and protocols were developed using estrogen in combination with cyclic progesterone or synthetic progestin given 10 to 14 days each month. Uterine cancer rates fell dramatically when cyclic progesterone was introduced. This is understandable, since progesterone is the natural mechanism by which the body sheds the endometrial lining each month.

In the 1990s, gynecologists began using daily progestins or progesterone in combination with oral estrogen and found they could usually eliminate the occurrence of the monthly period and still protect against uterine cancer. The use of daily progestin became the standard. In my experience, when used with topical estradiol, daily progesterone often did not eliminate periods and caused irregular bleeding. Unpredictable irregular bleeding is a nuisance to women so I resumed cyclic progesterone. Cyclic progesterone plus topical estradiol produces light, predictable monthly periods.

Progesterone Or Synthetic Progestin
Cyclic or Daily Use?

From the history lesson, you see we have gone from primarily using cyclic to daily use of progestins, but it seems we are now coming full circle. I believe there are compelling reasons to revisit this topic. The issues to consider: 1) whether progesterone/progestin should be given as a cyclic or a daily regimen, 2) whether to give progesterone or a synthetic progestin or 3) whether to give a very low-dose estrogen with no progesterone and do yearly pelvic sonograms. The only problem with the latter is ensuring that the woman on low-dose estrogen has an adequate estradiol level.

Daily use of progestins became the norm because it eliminated periods while still protecting against uterine cancer. However, WHI showed adverse risks of increased breast cancer, strokes and heart attacks from giving oral estrogens with daily *medroxyprogesterone* (MPA). Recent studies have implicated the continuous daily progestin since risks were less with estrogen alone. For more discussion on the risks of adding continuous daily progestins, see Chapter 21, *Risks of Adding Oral Progestins*. Since you can get the same protection against endometrial cancer from either cyclic or continuous progestin, taking a continuous progestin seems like a steep price to pay just to not have a period!

The adverse effect is probably not unique to MPA since a recent study comparing breast cancer risk by the type of HRT showed that all the regimens employing any synthetic progestin with an estrogen had an increased risk of breast cancer. The only regimen that had no increased risk of breast cancer was the group receiving estradiol plus progesterone. As more studies are done showing that progesterone has fewer risks than synthetic progestin, prescribing habits will have to change.

For the time being, as an advocate for my patients, I feel compelled to choose the safer regimen; That appears to be cyclic progesterone. Another reason for my decision is that cyclic progesterone is the "normal" way in which a woman's body produces progesterone. It makes good sense to choose a process and a hormone that has evolved over millions of years. Mother Nature does not make a lot of mistakes. We usually encounter fewer side effects when we respect the normal physiology of the human body. While cyclic progesterone is my preference if subsequent studies show that continuous progesterone is as safe as cyclic progesterone, then I will offer that choice to my patients.

I Have To Have Periods Again?

Menopausal women who previously had heavy, painful menstrual periods are often upset to learn that periods will return when they start HRT. However, the periods that occur from appropriately prescribed HRT are never heavy like the periods of premenopausal women. The heaviness of the period is related to the amount of estrogen you are taking. Premenopausal women produce markedly higher levels of estradiol that explains the heavier flow. An occasional woman will have a psychological aversion to the notion of having a monthly period again and for these women we respect their wishes and have them on daily progesterone that usually eliminates the occurrence of periods.

For those women who choose to take cyclic progesterone, this is how I explain the periods that accompany HRT. Estrogen and progesterone have a myriad of beneficial effects on every tissue in your body. One of these effects stimulates growth of the lining of the uterus that supports the sustaining of a pregnancy. Of course, a menopausal woman has no need for that effect on her uterus; but, it's part of the "total woman package" that occurs when you take estrogen. In order to receive the other beneficial effects you want from estrogen, you need to have a way in which to protect your uterine lining from excessive growth. The natural solution the female body has developed is the monthly shedding of the uterine lining in the form of a menstrual period. Without this cleansing of the uterus, you are subjecting yourself to an eight-fold increase in the risk of uterine cancer. This risk is easily eliminated with the right dose of progesterone.

With low doses of estrogen, the periods are much lighter than premenopausal periods. If periods are light, predictable, and have minimal cramping, most women accept them as a trade-off that protects their uterus against uterine cancer. The monthly period is a sign the uterine lining is being properly discharged each month. Heavy, painful periods are never acceptable. They're a sign of improper dosing of hormones or pathology within the uterus. This type of period should be further investigated with a *transvaginal ultrasound* (TVS).

TVS measures the lining of the uterus called the endometrial echo to check for signs of uterine cancer. If the lining is thickened it could be a sign of *hyperplasia,* a benign condition that sometimes precedes uterine cancer or it could have progressed to uterine cancer. In either case, a thickened uterine lining requires an endometrial biopsy, an office procedure to determine the cause of the thickening. If the biopsy shows no evidence of cancer, it likely represents hyperplasia, a benign overgrowth of tissue that is managed by adjusting the levels of estrogen and progesterone.

Despite seemingly normal monthly periods, I still recommend women on HRT undergo a yearly TVS of the uterus and ovaries. A thin uterine lining and small shrunken ovaries are reassuring signs that lessen the likelihood of endometrial or ovarian cancer. It is important to perform the TVS on day 5 or 6 of the menstrual cycle. The first day you bleed is day one of your menstrual cycle so this means the TVS is done just after a period has been completed. Logically, the uterine lining should be at its smallest just after a menstrual period.

Because a normal woman primarily produces progesterone only during the last two weeks of her menstrual cycle, it makes sense to give progesterone in this same cyclic pattern. If a woman has stopped her periods completely, a common practice is to add progesterone the first half of each calendar month. This makes it easier to remember when to take her progesterone. Periods generally occur within two days after the end of the progesterone phase. So in summary, the combination of estrogen and progesterone leads to the build-up of the uterine lining and stopping the progesterone initiates the shedding of the uterine lining as the menstrual flow.

When oral progesterone is given daily, in most women it interferes with the build-up of the uterine lining eventually leading to cessation of all menstrual bleeding in the first six months. However, about 20% of women on estrogen plus daily progesterone, may have unpredictable, bothersome bleeding and spotting requiring a daily pad or tampon indefinitely. While such bleeding is usually not heavy, most such women prefer to return to cyclic progesterone so they are not bothered by irregular and unpredictable bleeding the whole month.

PROGESTERONE PREPARATIONS

Pharmaceutical Oral and Vaginal Preparations

Pharmaceutical micronized oral progesterone is available as *Prometrium* and as a generic. A commonly used regimen in the US for oral progesterone is 200 mg given at bedtime for the first 12 days of each calendar month or 100 mg daily. The most carefully studied dosage protocol in a multi-center trial recommended 200 mg given for 12 days each month or 100 mg given for 25 days each month. Endometrial biopsies taken at six month intervals showed no evidence of uterine cancer in either group and the group receiving daily therapy eventually stopped having any periods.

I generally give 14 days of cyclic progesterone because it offers even more protection of the endometrium, plus it comes closer to mimicking the cyclic pattern of progesterone production that normally occurs in the body. For women who insist on not having periods, I will prescribe continuous progesterone.

Many women tolerate oral progesterone without any difficulty. A nice side benefit is that when given at bedtime, oral progesterone causes sedation; helpful if they have insomnia. However, women with gastrointestinal problems such as irritable bowel syndrome with either diarrhea or constipation may not tolerate oral progesterone. A few women get breast tenderness or other PMS symptoms from oral progesterone.

In either instance or if they do not have a menstrual period from oral progesterone, vaginal progesterone (**Prochieve** 4% or 8%, **Crinone** 4% or 8%, **Endometrim** 100 mg) is a good option. Vaginal progesterone delivers a higher level of progesterone directly to the uterus. To ensure adequate protection, I prescribe vaginal progesterone the first 14 days of each calendar month. Women on higher doses of topical estradiol, usually need 14 days of 8% vaginal progesterone to prevent the occurrence of heavy periods.

A study in menopausal women on estrogen showed that 91.9% of those receiving 4% cyclic vaginal progesterone for the first 12 days of each calendar month had predictable periods at six months. In another group on estrogen receiving 4% vaginal progesterone twice weekly throughout the month, 80.6% had cessation of periods by six months.

The package inserts for both *Prochieve* and *Crinone* suggest every other day use for 12 days but this is the dose for pre-menopausal women who have missed their periods and are not pregnant. In these women, this regimen of 4% progester-one serves as a "challenge" dose to reset their monthly cycles. In pregnant women with low progesterone, protocols of 8% vaginal progesterone in single or multiple doses are com-monly used to provide additional support to maintain their pregnancies. In perimenopausal women, vaginal progesterone can be very useful for controlling heavy menstrual bleeding sometimes seen in perimenopause.

Compounded Oral, Vaginal and Topical Progesterone

If a woman has an allergy to the peanut oil used in oral pro-gesterone, compounded oral progesterone can be prescribed. Compounded vaginal progesterone suppositories are also available. When cost is a major concern for a woman, com-pounded products are much less expensive than brand-name pharmaceutical products. Compounded topical progesterone creams are available but have the least degree of absorption and I do **not** recommend them. Because progesterone is so critical for protecting against uterine cancer, the poor absorption of topical progesterone cream is troubling. At the 2009 NAMS annual meeting, a clinical poster presentation reported two cases of endometrial cancer in women using estrogen with topical progesterone. As with any woman with an intact uterus, it is essential that a transvaginal sonogram be done yearly to ensure protection of the uterus against endometrial cancer.

PROGESTERONE PREPARATIONS

Oral Progesterone

Prometrium, 100 mg and 200 mg gel caps; also generic

Vaginal Progesterone

Crinone 4% and 8% vaginal cream in unit dose applicators
Endometrin 100 mg vaginal tablets

Topical Progesterone (Compounded) – Not recommended because of poor absorption

SYNTHETIC PROGESTIN PREPARATIONS

Oral Progestins

Medroxyprogesterone - *Provera* 2.5 mg, 5 mg and 10 mg tablets; also generic.

Norethindrone - *Aygestin* 5 mg tablets; also available as generic.

Intrauterine Device Progestin

An intrauterine device, **Mirena**, is inserted into the uterus by a healthcare provider. This device is designed to release a daily dose of 0.02 mg of levonorgestrel directly into the uterine lining. It is FDA-approved as a contraceptive but has been used "off-label" to protect the uterus in women receiving estrogen replacement therapy.

Off-Label Prescribing

Physicians can legally prescribe "off-label" medications if they see clinical merit. However, pharmaceutical companies are not allowed to promote these indications to physicians because they have not supplied the FDA with the necessary documentation to receive approval for this indication. Off-label prescribing more commonly occurs with older, generic drugs that no longer have patent protection. The pharmaceutical company has no financial incentive to submit studies to the FDA. However, when physicians see clinical effectiveness, such medications continue to be prescribed.

Topical Progestin Estrogen Combinations, See pp. 203-4

Chapter 26

Testosterone
Achieving a delicate balance

When a woman goes through menopause and her ovaries stop producing estrogen and progesterone, the pituitary responds by increasing FSH, a hormone from the pituitary gland that has regulated these hormones throughout her reproductive life. However, when all the eggs have been depleted, no further estrogen or progesterone can be produced. Nonetheless, the pituitary which is "hard-wired" to respond to low estrogen, continues to make increasingly higher levels of FSH. An elevated FSH is a diagnostic marker indicating menopause has occurred. Testosterone production occurs not from the eggs, but from different cells in the ovary which continue to function in the postmenopausal ovary. Such increases in FSH leads to increased testosterone production. Testosterone can also be produced in fat cells and in the adrenal gland. A postmenopausal woman with even normal testosterone in the presence of deficient estrogen often develops facial hair and acne. This explains why older women without HRT often develop facial hair and a deepening of their voice. Care should be taken to restore therapeutic levels of estradiol and progesterone before giving testosterone. Restoring therapeutic estrogen and progesterone lowers FSH resulting in a decline in testosterone production. However, FSH levels never return to levels seen in premenopausal women.

Testosterone replacement is especially important in younger women who undergo surgical menopause. They will often have marked decline in libido and sexual dysfunction and may also develop urinary frequency and incontinence. Some studies suggest testosterone in the presence of estrogen and progesterone has a protective effect on the breast and may decrease breast cancer risk.

On the other hand, studies in premenopausal and postmenopausal women (on no HRT) who had naturally occurring elevated testosterone showed that testosterone is associated with an increased risk of breast cancer. In the *Study of Women's Health Across the Nation* (SWAN), a longitudinal 9-year-study of 949 menopausal women on no HRT reported that testosterone predominance increases the incidence of metabolic syndrome. *Metabolic syndrome* is a name for a group of risk factors that increases your risk of heart disease and diabetes. Typically, people have elevations in blood pressure and fasting blood sugar, increased obesity around their waist and/or low HDL. In another study of 344 menopausal women ages 65-98, those with the highest levels of testosterone were three times more likely to have heart disease and metabolic syndrome than those women with lower testosterone levels.

Such studies point out the importance of respecting the normal physiology of the body. Testosterone is best prescribed after the woman is on adequate estrogen. **Since testosterone can be produced by menopausal ovaries and the adrenal glands, deficient levels should be confirmed with an accurate assay that measures free testosterone levels before prescribing testosterone.** Excessive testosterone replacement can cause facial hair, acne and loss of scalp hair and such symptoms are easily avoided by subsequent monitoring of blood levels.

TESTOSTERONE BLOOD ASSAYS

Because women's levels of testosterone are one-tenth that of men, it is important to use a test that accurately measures testosterone at the lower end of the scale. The most accurate "gold standard" is the free testosterone by equilibrium dialysis. Normal free testosterone is generally 0.4 to 0.8 ng/dl (40-80 pg/dl) but may vary depending on the reference range for your lab. A baseline blood free testosterone to confirm deficiency and follow-up testing 3 months after starting testosterone replacement is advisable.

TESTOSTERONE PREPARATIONS

There are two commercially available oral preparations for women which contain testosterone: *Estratest* and *Estratest-HS* (half strength). *Estratest* contains 1.25 mg of esterified estrogens and 2.5 mg of methyltestosterone while the HS formula contains half of each of these hormones. While these products are not FDA approved for sexual function, some physicians prescribe them in women with a low libido. I do not prescribe these hormones because as oral hormones, they carry higher risks as previously mentioned in Chapter 20 - *Risks From Oral Estrogen*. I also have not found them effective in improving libido.

Testosterone is commercially available for men and is marketed as **Androgel** and **Testim**, which are both topical gel preparations. These preparations can be used in small amounts ranging from 0.25 ml to 0.5 ml applied daily which represents a delivery dose of 0.25 mg and 0.5 mg respectively. *Testim* is probably the easier to use because it comes in a small tube that can be resealed. Start with a small pea-sized amount applied to the inner wrist each morning. One tube should last a woman for about six weeks.

Chapter 27

Monitoring blood hormone levels
And why it's important

Many women who initially see me for menopause have never had their estradiol level checked. Their previous physician may have diagnosed menopause with an elevated FSH, but usually no further tests are done. I'd like to go through various reasons why I believe it is important to monitor estradiol levels.

1. ESTROGEN IS A TWO-EDGED SWORD

I describe estrogen as a two-edged sword because it can be both protective and harmful depending on how your body uses it and on the amounts and duration of estrogen exposure. Endogenous estrogen refers to the levels of estradiol that a woman's own body produces before menopause. Early in the book I outlined how estrogen is essential to many cellular functions throughout the body. In Chapter 22 - *Risks of NOT Taking Estrogen*, I listed the many symptoms and degenerative consequences that can result from a low estrogen state.

On the other hand, estrogen excess throughout a woman's life is associated with increased risks of cancer. An increased risk of breast cancer is associated with longer exposure to endogenous estrogen, i.e. early menarche (starting your periods at an early age) and later menopause. Higher estrogen states seen with obesity increase the risk of breast cancer even more. Studies show women with a body mass index (BMI) over 35 have a twenty-fold increased risk of endometrial cancer.

Estrogen, estrone and testosterone can be produced from fat cells in obese postmenopausal women. These obese women also have lower production of a substance in the blood called *sex hormone binding globulin* (SHBG). SHBG serves as a carrier protein for storing estrogen in the blood. Lower levels of SHBG results in higher levels of available estrogen that thereby increases their estrogen exposure. In the Nurses' Health Study of a subset of women on no HRT, an increased risk of breast cancer was seen in women with the highest endogenous estradiol compared to those with the lowest estradiol. A similar increased risk was seen in women on no HRT with the highest endogenous level of testosterone. However, in women on HRT with low testosterone, studies show that adding testosterone can be beneficial in lessening the risk of breast cancer.

These potentially protective and harmful effects of estrogen go back to the basic tenet of any hormone - adverse symptoms can occur with deficiency or excess while optimal function develops with the right level. I see this as an affirmation of the need to respect the balance among the different sex hormones. Monitoring estradiol and testosterone blood levels enables us to prevent a deficient state while guarding against excess levels. This is a standard practice when physicians prescribe thyroid hormone. Why should it be any different for estrogen and testosterone?

2. VARIABILITY OF TOPICAL ABSORPTION

While levels are consistent within a given individual, tremendous variability in the efficiency of absorption can be found from one woman to another and this constitutes another reason to measure blood levels. In a study of women given identical doses of topical estradiol there was considerable variation in blood levels with estradiol increases above baseline differing as much as 90 pg/ml from one woman to another. Studies have even shown differences in absorption when changing women from one patch to a different brand of the same dose. Despite such variations, absorption of topical estradiol is more stable and consistent than oral estradiol which peaks at 4 to 5 hours and is non detectable by 8 to 10 hours.

This phenomenon of variable absorption with topical patches,gels and creams has been documented in numerous studies. Importantly, estradiol blood levels tend to be consistent within a given woman once appropriate levels are achieved and frequent dosage changes are not generally required. Annual monitoring of estradiol blood levels is generally adequate to ensure therapeutic levels. With increasing age of the woman, drug metabolism may be slower, requiring dose reduction to prevent excess estradiol levels.

Since I routinely monitor blood estradiol levels, I have seen such variation in topical absorption in the thousands of women I have managed. This may also explain why some women who first start topical estradiol sometimes give up saying "it doesn't work" and they switch to pills. Since you have learned of the lower risks from topical estradiol, it is worthwhile to persist in finding a topical product that works for you. In my clinical experience of managing over 100,000 female patient visits, I've found very few women who could not be managed with topical estradiol.

In general, thin women require higher estradiol doses while obese women with endogenous stores of estrogen in fat generally can be managed with a lower dose. Higher climate temperature in summer months may increase the need for higher doses of topical estrogen especially in women who are outdoors a lot and are very physically active. Women who take long hot baths will likely reduce estrogen absorption from estradiol patches because the hot water leaches estradiol from the patch. Taking showers does not have this effect. If a woman insists on long, hot, baths, she is best managed with topical gels and creams.

When a pharmaceutical drug is developed, in order to receive FDA approval, the manufacturer must show proof that their product has effectiveness and achieves significant blood levels. The pharmacology term for this is the *"drug-response curve."* Studies are done to establish the optimal dose that will achieve certain blood levels and the desired therapeutic effect with the least adverse side effects.

3. YOU CAN'T JUST GO BY "HOW YOU FEEL!"

I strongly endorse monitoring estradiol and testosterone blood levels to ensure appropriate dosage and effectiveness of hormone therapy. Monitoring estradiol levels in thousands of women since 1986 has led me to develop more precise hormone regimens producing blood levels comparable to a low physiologic range. As noted earlier, monitoring blood levels is especially important with topical therapy. Most postmenopausal women who see me initially have NEVER had their estrogen level checked!

Early heart disease and osteoporosis are both consequences of low estrogen and have no symptoms in many women. Hot flashes eventually go away in many women even without taking estrogen. Dosing hormones simply by "how you feel" is an archaic notion and other hormones like thyroid hormone and growth hormone are never dosed that way! It is time for menopause management to come into the 21st century and not be treated like a stepchild among other hormone deficiencies. A few lucky women go through menopause and never have hot flashes but this can be a mixed blessing. If you don't have symptoms, you're less likely to seek help. However, even without symptoms, you may still be at risk for the degenerative consequences of low estrogen.

For insidious problems like osteoporosis or heart disease, there are usually no symptoms until the woman has a fracture or heart attack. If estrogen dosage for such women is determined simply by "how they feel", we may be giving them an inadequate dose and putting them at increased risk. Objective measurement of blood estradiol ensures adequacy of dosage. Studies have shown a protective effect on bones from fairly low doses of estrogen. In one study of postmenopausal women treated with estrogen alone, those with higher estradiol levels had less progression of subclinical atherosclerosis on CIMT than those with lower estradiol. Recall that CIMT is an ultrasound measurement of the thickness of the two inner layers (the intima and media) of the carotid arteries that the *American Heart Association* recommends as the best way to screen for early risk of heart disease or stroke. I routinely rely on CIMT to assist me in assessing these risks in my patients.

In general, creams and gels produce lower blood estradiol levels ranging from 9.8 to 30 pg/ml that are similar to the lower doses of estradiol patches. The highest estradiol blood levels are achieved with the 0.1 mg estradiol patches and are typically in the range of 80 pg/ml.

More studies need to be done to determine the optimal level that protects us from the consequences of low estrogen while avoiding the adverse effects that may occur with the higher doses of estrogen. For the time being, a reasonable approach is to give the lowest estrogen dose that relieves symptoms and still falls within the lower physiologic range for a premeno-pausal woman.

4. IMPORTANCE OF ACCURATE BLOOD ASSAYS

When measuring estradiol levels it is very important that an assay be utilized which has the ability to detect the very low levels present in post-menopausal women. The estradiol assay used in fertility practices for women undergoing ovulation induction or in vitro fertilization is not appropriate. An assay with sensitivity at the low end of the scale is required to moni-tor estradiol therapy in menopausal women. The assay should be capable of measuring less than 1.5 ng/dL of estradiol or less than 1.0 pg/ml of free estradiol. Similarly for free testosterone, assays that utilize equilibrium dialysis are the most accurate at detecting the lower levels of testosterone seen in women.

When I first see a female patient, I may check estradiol blood levels several times in the first few months while adjusting their dosage. Once the levels are stable, I check them once a year unless symptoms develop or there is another dosage change. Since postmenopausal ovaries often continue to prod-uct testosterone, it is important to document low testosterone levels **before** prescribing testosterone.

For a woman with an intact uterus, withdrawal periods on cyclic progesterone and a normal yearly TVS, there is less need to monitor progesterone. "Withdrawal periods" is the medi-cal term given to the monthly menstrual flow occurring in postmenopausal women prescribed estrogen with cyclic pro-gesterone. When a woman is perimenopausal and still having periods, progesterone levels on day 21 of her menstrual cycle are a useful indication of her endogenous progesterone. If low, adding progesterone therapy may improve symptoms of heavy bleeding, PMS or insomnia.

5. SALIVARY HORMONE TESTING IS NOT RELIABLE

Many women ask me about salivary hormone tests. While dependent on the accuracy of the testing laboratory, you can measure hormone levels of estradiol, progesterone and testosterone in saliva. However, an important reason for measuring hormones is to be able to determine the optimal dose of the hormone preparation. Salivary hormone tests are notoriously unreliable for this purpose. Numerous studies have shown inconsistent and skewed results with the use of salivary hormone testing in women on HRT. That's why I utilize blood hormone testing.

Seeing the big picture
& the cycle of life

Afterword

Where Do We Stand Now?

Although the debate over the safety of hormone replacement still rages in the press, it appears some semblance of common sense is beginning to be heard. Yes, we need more confirming studies, but today's women - myself included - cannot be put on hold and forced to wait another 10 to 20 years until all of the definitive studies have been completed. As with so many other issues in medicine, physicians have to use their best clinical judgment based on the information available now. Each woman needs to make these decisions with input from her own physician.

After all my years of practice, I still believe we should try to mimic the normal human physiology whenever possible. That's why I use topical over oral hormones, cyclic over continuous progesterone, and natural over synthetic hormones whenever possible. My goal with any patient is to give the lowest dose of hormone that corrects her symptoms and still gives her therapeutic levels of her natural hormones. However, no prescription drug, including hormones, is without side effects or totally free of risks. That's why it requires a prescription: so your physician can safely develop a hormone program that is monitored and takes into account all your medical concerns. Because the endocrinologist is the definitive hormone specialist, it's ideal to have bioidentical HRT prescribed and monitored by an endocrinologist. However, there is a shortage of endocrinologists who treat menopause. For that reason it is important to seek out a gynecologist, internist or family practitioner who has acquired expertise in treating menopause with bioidentical hormone therapy and to take responsibility for educating yourself about menopause and its related conditions.

The Economic Costs and Their Implications

At this time in our nation's history we are faced with ever mounting costs in the health care system. I have stated the importance of patient education and individual accountability for achieving good health. I believe that if the women now taking oral hormones would change to topical HRT, and if 80% of women were taking HRT instead of 20%, this would translate into better health for women and result in enormous savings in health care dollars. It is beyond the scope of this book to analyze the cost savings if 80% of menopausal women were taking topical estrogen; there are multiple variables affecting each related condition. For example bone loss can occur in a woman on estrogen if she is taking inadequate calcium or vitamin D.

I have listed the health care costs of some more common disorders that occur in a low estrogen state. Providing safer, preventive therapy that improves quality of life and has potential to save health care costs should be a goal for all patients and the healthcare system.

Osteoporosis

The annual health care expenditure for osteoporosis fractures in U.S. women over 45 years old in 1995 was $11 billion including inpatient hospital, nursing home, and outpatient care. By 2005, according to the *National Osteoporosis Foundation*, that figure rose to $15.2 billion for all osteoporotic fractures in U.S. women.

Heart Disease

In 2009, heart disease in women is expected to cost more than $152 billion, including health care services, medications and lost productivity.

Alzheimer's Disease and Dementia

The direct cost to Medicare and Medicaid for treating women with Alzheimer's and dementia, and the indirect costs to business of employees who are caregivers for these Alzheimer patients, is more than $75 billion per year. This figure is expected to increase as the population ages. Medicare costs for Alzheimer's patients are three times higher than other conditions of Medicare recipients.

Making the Most of the Post-Menopausal Years

The onset of menopause saddens many women because they fear the age-related changes to come and see it as a loss of their femininity. It is my mission to help you see menopause as simply the next stage in the normal cycle of life. However, unlike our grandmothers, we do not need to passively accept deterioration of our minds and bodies. Yes, we will all die of something eventually, but there are many proactive things we can now do to soften the impact of aging and increase our enjoyment of life. Bioidentical HRT, exercise, healthy eating, not smoking, plus other self-care measures play a major role in decreasing the disability of aging.

At this time, less than 20 percent of postmenopausal women use HRT, presumably because of the perceived risk and lack of knowledge of available treatments. It should be clear now that millions of these women are suffering needlessly from the symptoms of menopause. We have discussed what is happening to the reproductive system during menopause, especially the dramatically decreased levels of estrogen. We have examined the controversy regarding estrogen replacement, have acknowledged that there is some risk, and have contrasted those risks with the risks of no hormone therapy. Choosing topical delivery systems and avoiding continuous synthetic progestins can often reduce risks.

In my view, failing to provide patients HRT when they are in such desperate need is failing to honor a physician's primary responsibility - to do no harm. In this area, to do nothing is to do harm.

Seeing Ourselves in Nature

The beauty of living into older age comes when you achieve a level of maturity that enables you to see and feel your connection to the cycle of life. You come to see the wonders of the natural world with new eyes that are both knowing and childlike in their appreciation. It's a poignant moment of awareness that gives you a glimpse of the intricate, orderly balance of nature and how you fit into the cycle of life.

I recall the times my family and I have traveled to the *Muir Woods* in California. The great redwoods rise like ancient cathedrals into clouds white as the corner of a child's eye. It is here in the deep Gothic silences that I realize once again that we are not apart from nature but an integral part of nature. We are made of the same elements as the redwood, the eagle, the mountain, and even the stars. So much of our design resembles the design of other life forms. Under a microscope, human epidermis resembles the bark of a maple tree; the spiral of the inner ear chamber is identical to a snail shell, white blood cells look like pollen and blood vessels resemble the veins in a leaf. The patterns that unfold in our bodies are the same patterns that are found on the shells of creatures of the sea or in the petals of a flower.

There are distant nebulas in the cosmos shaped exactly like the spiral ladders of DNA, the basic component of human life. What other word could define the elegant double-helix spiral of DNA better than "perfection"? Philosophers have defined perfection as "a state of completeness, flawlessness." Aristotle wrote: *"That which is perfect contains all the required parts, which is so good that nothing of its kind could be better. Perfection is that which has attained its purpose."* I often think the design of the human body approaches perfection in form and function. It is a perfect machine made up of many complicated parts.

How different the running of such a machine from that of one imperfectly constructed and unequally balanced. One seldom needs repair, the other frequently. Given proper care and nutrients, the human body is capable of sustaining and healing itself. Of all the wondrous things God has made, none compare to the elegant symmetry, the interlocking complexity, the natural beauty and magical power of the body-mind of man and the body-mind of woman.

Consider the extraordinary miracle of the developing embryo in the womb where we can actually see the beating heart in a fetus the size of a lima bean. Barely two weeks after conception, cells within the embryo are reproducing at a rate of 250,000 times per minute. By the seventh month, the wiring in the brain has some 10 trillion connections some thousands of miles long. The human body is a marvel of engineering, far more complex and awe-inspiring than any man-made creation. Its beauty and strength reside not in one part or another, but in the harmonious interplay of the whole. Consider the miracle of the human heart. The heart beats about 100,000 times a day. At age 70, it will have beat at least 2.5 billion times, pumping approximately a million gallons of blood carrying oxygen and nutrients through a system of tubes that, if laid end to end, would reach more than three times around the world. What other machine can function so robustly, so perfectly, under various conditions, for so long? Consider all this and know that you alone have been entrusted with the care of this electronics and chemistry and mechanics and elaborate engineering - this clockwork of life.

This is the gift we have been given. And now, after menopause, we are given 30 more years to care for it. To some extent, we can slow down the effects of aging by replacing deficient hormones and giving more attention to self-care. Your physician can provide you with hormones that facilitate the balance required by the endocrine system. However you can do so much more to amplify the physician's efforts when you become part of the solution. When you become accountable for your own health, you and your physician become powerful allies.

Acknowledgements

This book has been a long, painstaking three-year process that I've written while running a full-time, busy, clinical practice. There are many, many people who have helped me along the way.

I want to extend a special thanks to Dr. Daniel R. Mishell, Professor Emeritus at the University of Southern California School of Medicine for his guidance in helping me with the writing of this book. Dr. Mishell is a preeminent academic researcher who was the first to describe the hormone pattern of the female menstrual cycle in 1971. I met him at a lecture he gave on menopausal hormone therapy in May 2009 and we have had a collegial, personal, e-mail correspondence since then. He graciously reviewed my manuscript and gave me constructive comments that improved the book. To me a sign of a great physician is his willingness to be a mentor and share his wisdom and knowledge with other physicians.

I would like to thank my husband and Practice Administrator, Gordon Blocker for his leadership and strategic planning in the design and marketing of this project. From his years of experience as a successful film, video and interactive producer/director, he directed a team of talented consultants to craft the vision for the company brand we are today. Our partnership is complementary in so many ways.

My daughter, Afton M. Johnson, soon to be a physician herself, assisted me in editing and giving me moral support and encouragement.

I wish to thank the following consultants for their outstanding contributions and sage advice:

Front & Back Cover Artwork:
Maria Rendon

Book Cover, Layout & Chart Illustrations:
Glenn Hadsall

Eyesong Publishing:
Gordon Blocker

Institute Branding and Design Creative Director:
Les Kerr

Branding and Website Team:
Glenn Hadsall, Les Baker and Mark DeMoss

Manuscript and Editing Contributions:
Marshall Riggan, Poppy Sundeen, Bruce Anderson,
Afton Johnson, Kim Young and Manisha H. Maskay, Ph.D.

Strategic Marketing Concepts:
Gordon Blocker, Barbara Steckler-Friedlander, Kim Young and
Bruce Anderson

Marketing Graphics and Flash Design:
Glenn Hadsall

Legal Consultant:
Mark Walker, Esq

Portrait Photographer:
Kent Barker

Social Marketing Consultants:
Nicole Scaglione, Jennifer Browning and Kim Young

Eyesong Publishing Logo Design:
Cam Pietralunga

Spiritual Guidance:
Dr. Ed Pauley and Anne Holland

Website Development & eBook Technical Consultants:
William Ballard, Glenn Hadsall and Kovid Goyal

Facebook Focus Group:
Marilyn Reiswerg Descours, Sally Hill Maslansky, Paula Trost, Irene Sheppard, Patsy DeSalvo, Alison Oliver Kelly, Denese Midkiff Kiecke, Andrea Perez Robinson, Marlee Bisbey, Sarita Bullard Oerling, Janice McInnis, R.N. and Becky Odom McAllister

IEPM Office Staff:
Kathleen Hartley, my lead research assistant and Nancy Valerin, Susan Lampley, John Huddleston and my nursing staff who all helped me maintain a busy practice while writing the book.

I want to thank Mark Walker, a prominent business attorney and patient, who gave me very helpful comments and even did a survey of the women in his office asking their opinion about certain sections to improve clarity and relevance.

Many patients have read my manuscript and given me valuable suggestions as I have utilized the manuscript as a patient education tool. In alphabetical order, these include: Bill and Susan Casner, Catherine Crier, Hiya Hoffman, Joni Lamb,

Sandra Magnuson, Pam Minick, Natasha Naquin, Cindy Waldrip and Mark Walker.

A special thanks to Dr. Bradley Bale, an assistant clinical professor at Texas Tech School of Medicine, specializing in cardiovascular prevention. Brad is a colleague, a friend and a mentor. He and Amy Doneen, MSN, ARNP, founded the Heart Attack and Stroke Prevention Clinic in Spokane, Washington. Their work led to the development of the *Bale/Doneen Method,* a powerful model for early detection and treatment of the root causes that lead to heart disease, strokes and diabetes. Combining their system with pharmaceutical bioidentical hormones has enabled me to provide more comprehensive care to my patients. Their approach to prevention of these diseases has become an integral component of the **Johnson Menopause Method**™.

The following doctors kindly provided assistance in their areas of expertise: Daniel Mishell, Jr., Professor Emeritus, USC School of Medicine; Donald Massaro, M.D., Professor of Medicine, Georgetown School of Medicine; Dan Silverman, M.D., PhD., Associate Professor, UCLA School of Medicine; Alan Altman, M.D., Aspen, Colorado; Mary Ann Mehn, PhD. and MK Goldstein, PhD., both of MammaCare, Gainesville, Florida and Ellen Lokkegaard M.D., PhD. of Copenhagen, Denmark.

I want to thank the many patients who have given me the honor and privilege of entrusting me with their health care. Seeing their progress and transformation has been gratifying and exhilarating. When I encounter a problem, it motivates me to further expand my knowledge to find solutions. It is a gradual, evolving process that continually sharpens ones clinical skills.

And I thank God for giving me the curiosity to pursue the joy of ongoing learning and for allowing me to use that knowledge to improve the health of women.

External Links

Outliving Your Ovaries
http://www.OutlivingYourOvaries.com

The Institute of Endocrinology and Preventive Medicine
http://www.DrMarinaJohnson.com

The Dr. Marina Johnson Facebook Site
http://www.Facebook.com/DrMarinaJohnson

The Dr. Marina Johnson on YouTube
http://www.YouTube.com/DrMarinaJohnsonTV

The Dr. Marina Johnson on Twitter
http://Twitter.com/DrMarinaJohnson

The Dr. Marina Johnson Store
http://www.DrMarinaJohnsonStore.com

Eyesong Publishing
http://www.EyesongPublishing.com

References

Chapter 2 - Introduction

1. Russell, LB, "Prevention and Medicare costs," *New England Journal of Medicine*, vol. 339 (1998): pp 1158-1160.
2. Hill, JW, Futterman, R, *et al*, "Alzheimer's disease and related dementias increase costs of comorbidities in managed Medicare," *Neurology*, vol. 58 (2002): pp 62-70.
3. Daviglus, ML, Liu, K, Pirzada, A, *et al*, "Cardiovascular risk profile earlier in life and Medicare costs in the last year of life," *Archives Internal Medicine*, vol. 165 (2005): pp 1028-1034.
4. Lubitz, JD and Riley, GF, "Trends in Medicare payments in the last year of life," *New England Journal of Medicine*, vol. 328 (1993): pp 1092-1096.

Chapter 4 - Principles influencing my approach to medicine

1. Holman, H, "Chronic disease - The need for a new clinical education," *Journal of the American Medical Association*, vol. 292 no. 9 (2004): pp 1057-1059.
2. Green, S, (Letter to the Editor) "Medical education and chronic disease," *Journal of the American Medical Association*, vol. 292, no. 24 (2004): p 2974.
3. Kirkegaard, M, (Letter to the Editor) "Medical education and chronic disease," *Journal of the American Medical Association*, vol. 292 no. 24 (2004): p 2974.
4. Morioka-Douglas, N, (Letter to the Editor) "Medical education and chronic disease," *Journal of the American Medical Association*, vol. 292, no. 24 (2004): p 2975.
5. Brehm, JG, (Letter to the Editor) "Medical education and chronic disease," *Journal of the American Medical Association*, vol. 292 no. 24 (2004): p 2975.

6. Karha, J and Topol, EJ, "The sad story of Vioxx and what we should learn from it," *Cleveland Clinic Journal of Medicine*, vol. 71, no.12 (2004): pp 933-939.

7. Brett, KM and Chong, Y, "Hormone replacement therapy: Knowledge and use in the United States," Hyattsville, Maryland: National Institutes of Health, *National Center for Health Statistics* (2001).

Chapter 6 - The symphony within - the endocrine system

1. Kronenberg HM, Melmed S, Polonsky KS, *et al*, (Editors): *Williams Textbook of Endocrinology*, 11th edition, (2007) Chapter 16, The Physiology and Pathology of the Female Reproductive Axis.

Chapter 7 - Hormones of the reproductive system

1. Mishell, DR Jr., Nakamura, RM, Crosignani, PG, *et al*, "Serum gonadotropin and steroid patterns during the normal menstrual cycle," *American Journal of Obstetrics & Gynecology*, vol. 111, no.1 (1971): pp 60-65.

2. Dubey, RK and Jackson, EK, "Estrogen-induced cardiorenal protection: Potential cellular, biochemical, and molecular mechanisms," *American Journal of Physiology - Renal Physiology*, vol. 280 (2001): pp 365-388.

3. Speroff, L and Fritz, MA (Editors), *Clinical Gynecologic Endocrinology and Infertility*, 7th Edition, (2005) Lippincott, Williams & Wilkins, pp 25-44.

4. Chen, Z, Yuhanna, IS, *et al*, "Estrogen receptor alpha mediates the nongenomic activation of endothelial nitric oxide synthase by estrogen," *The Journal of Clinical Investigation*, vol. 103(3) (1999): pp 401-406.

5. Helguero, LA, Faulds, MH, Gustafsson JA, *et al*, "Estrogen receptors alpha (ER-alpha) and beta (ER-beta) differentially regulate proliferation and apoptosis of the normal murine mammary epithelial cell line HC11", *Oncogene*, vol. 24 (2005): pp 6605-6616.

6. Rissman, EF, "Roles of oestrogen receptors alpha and beta in behavioral neuroendocrinology: beyond yin/yang," *Journal of Neuroendocrinology*, vol. 20(6) (2008): pp 873-879.

7. Walsh, BA, Mullick, AE, *et al*, "17 beta-estradiol acts separately on the LDL particle and artery wall to reduce LDL accumulation," *The Journal of Lipid Research*, vol. 41(2000): pp 134-141.

8. Dubey, RK and Jackson, EK, "Genome and hormones: gender differences in physiology invited review: cardiovascular protective effects of 17 beta-estradiol metabolites," *Journal of Applied Physiology*, vol. 91 (2001): pp 1868-1883.

9. Miller, VM and Duckles, SP, "Vascular actions of estrogens: functional implications," *Pharmacological Reviews* vol. 60 (2008): pp 210-241.

10. Zelinski-Wooten, MB; Hess DL, *et al*, "Administration of an aromatase inhibitor during the late follicular phase of gonadotropin-treated cycles in rhesus monkeys: effects on follicle development, oocyte maturation, and subsequent luteal function," *Journal of Clinical Endocrinology and Metabolism*, vol. 76(4) (1993): pp 988-95.

11. McEwen, BS, "Gonadal hormone receptors on the developing and adult brain: relationship to the regulatory phenotype," *Fetal Neuroendocrinology*, Perinatology Press, Ithaca, 1984.

12. Colvard, DS, Eriksen, EF, *et al*, "Identification of androgen receptors in normal human osteoblast-like cells," *Proceedings of the National Academy of Sciences of the United States of America*, vol. 86(3) (1989): pp 854-7.

13. Hutchinson, KA, "Androgens and sexuality," *American Journal of Medicine*, vol. 98(1A) (1995): pp 111S-115S.

Chapter 10 - The reproductive years

1. Treloar, AE, Boynton, RE, *et al*, "Variation of the human menstrual cycle through reproductive life," *International Journal of Fertility and Women's Medicine*, vol. 12 (1967): p 77.

2. Adams, Hillard PJ, "Menstruation in adolescents: what's normal, what's not," *Annals of New York Academy of Science*, vol. 1135 (2008): pp 29-35.

3. Fortner, KB and Wallach, EE, *The Johns Hopkins Manual of Gynecology and Obstetrics,* 3rd edition (2006): pp 445-6.
4. Ragucci, KR, "Treatment of female sexual dysfunction," *The Annals of Pharmacotherapy,* vol. 37(4) (2003): pp 546-555.
5. Panzer, C, Wise, S, Fantini, G, *et al,* "Impact of oral contraceptives on sex hormone-binding globulin and androgen levels: a retrospective study in women with sexual dysfunction," *Journal of Sexual Medicine,* vol. 3(1) (2006): pp 104-113.
6. Sherman, BM and Korenman, SG, "Hormonal characteristics of the human menstrual cycle throughout reproductive life," *The Journal of Clinical Investigation,* vol. 55(4) (1975): pp 699-706.
7. Stanford, JB, White, GL, Hatasaka H, "Timing intercourse to achieve pregnancy: current evidence," *Obstetrics and Gynecology,* vol. 100(6) (2002): pp 1333-41.
8. Lidegaard, O, *et al,* "Hormonal contraception and risk of venous thromboembolism: national follow-up study," *British Medical Journal,* vol. 339 (2009): pp b2890.
9. van Hylckama, Vlieg A, *et al,* "The venous thrombotic risk of oral contraceptives, effects of oestrogen dose and progestogen type: results of the MEGA case-control study," *British Medical Journal,* vol. 339 (2009): pp b2921.
10. Adams, Hillard PJ, "Menstruation in adolescents: what's normal?," *The Medscape Journal of Medicine,* vol. 10(12) (2008): p 295.

Chapter 12 - The symptoms of menopause - is it hot in here?

1. Beckman, M., "All fat is not created equal," *Science of Aging Knowledge Environment,* vol. 2002(41) (2002): p nw 143.
2. Carlson, CL, Cushman, M, Enright, PL, *et al,* "Hormone replacement therapy is associated with higher FEV1 in elderly women," *American Journal of Respiratory and Critical Care Medicine,* vol. 163 (2001): pp 423-428.
3. Massaro, D and Massaro, GD, "Estrogen regulates pulmonary alveolar formation, loss, and regeneration in mice," *American Journal of Physiology - Lung Cellular and Molecular Physiology,* vol. 287 (2004): pp L1154-L1159.

4. D'Elia, HF, Larsen A, Mattsson LA, *et al,* "Influence of hormone replacement therapy on disease progression and bone mineral density in rheumatoid arthritis," *The Journal of Rheumatology,* vol. 30(7) (2003): pp 1456-1463.

5. Massaro, GD, Mortola, JP and Massaro, D, "Estrogen modulates the dimensions of the lung's gas-exchange surface area and alveoli in female rats," *American Journal of Physiology - Lung Cellular and Molecular Physiology,* vol. 270 (1996): pp L110-L114.

6. D'Elia, HF, Mattsson, LA, Ohlsson C, *et al,* "Hormone replacement therapy in rheumatoid arthritis is associated with lower serum levels of soluble IL-6 receptor and higher insulin-like growth factor 1," *Arthritis Research and Therapy,* vol. 5(4) (2003): pp R202-R209.

Chapter 13 - Natural menopause

1. Grodin, JM, *et al,* "Source of estrogen production in postmenopausal women," *Journal of Clinical Endocrinology and Metabolism,* vol. 36(2) (1973): pp 207-214.

Chapter 14 - Surgical menopause - under the knife

1. Domchek, SM, Rebbeck, TR, "Prophylactic oophorectomy in women at increased cancer risk," *Current Opinion in Obstetrics and Gynecology,* vol. 19(1) (2007): pp 27-30.

2. Parker, WH, *et al,* "Ovarian conservation at the time of hysterectomy for benign disease," *Obstetrics and Gynecology,* vol. 106(2) (2005): pp 219-226.

3. Parish, H.M., *et al,* "Time interval from castration in premenopausal women to development of excessive coronary atherosclerosis," *American Journal of Obstetrics and Gynecology,* vol. 99(2) (1967): pp 155-162.

4. Colditz, G.A., *et al,* "Menopause and the risk of coronary heart disease in women," *New England Journal of Medicine,* vol. 316(18) (1987): pp 1105-1110.

5. Das, N, Kay, VJ, and Mahmood, TA, "Current knowledge of risks and benefits of prophylactic oophorectomy at hysterectomy for benign disease in United Kingdom and Republic of Ireland," *European Journal of Obstetrics and Gynecology and Reproductive Biology*, vol. 109 (2003): pp 76-79.

6. Labrie, F, *et al*, "Endocrine and intracrine sources of androgens in women: inhibition of breast cancer and other roles," *Endocrine Reviews*, vol. 24(2) (2003): pp 152-182.

7. Somboonporn, W, and Davis, SR, "Postmenopausal testosterone therapy and breast cancer risk," *Maturitas*, vol. 49 (2004): pp 267-270.

8. Rivera, CM, *et al*, "Increased cardiovascular mortality after early bilateral oophorectomy," *Menopause*, vol. 16 (2009): p 15.

9. Parker, WH and Manson, JE, "Oophorectomy and cardiovascular mortality: is there a link?," *Menopause*, vol. 16 (2009): p 1.

10. Rebbeck, TR, *et al*, "Meta-analysis of risk reduction estimates associated with risk-reducing salpingo-oophorectomy in BRCA1 or BRCA2 mutation carriers," *Journal of National Cancer Institute*, vol. 101 (2009): p 80.

11. Greene, MH and Mai, PL, "What have we learned from risk-reducing salpingo-oophorectomy?," *Journal of National Cancer Institute*, vol. 101 (2009): p 70.

12. Parker, WH, *et al*, "Ovarian conservation at the time of hysterectomy and long-term health outcomes in the Nurses' Health Study," *Obstetrics and Gynecology*, vol. 113 (2009): p 1027.

13. Thurston RC, Abstract S-8, presented at the 20th Annual North American Menopause Society Meeting; Sept. 30-Oct. 3, 2009; San Diego

14. Thurston RC, Sutton-Tyrrell K, Everson-Rose SA, *et al*, "Hot flashes and subclinical cardiovascular disease," *Circulation*, vol 118 (2008): pp 1234-1240.

15. Johnson DB, Dwyer KM, Stanczyk FZ, *et al*, "The relationship of menopausal status and rapid menopausal transition with carotid intima-media thickness progress in women: a report from the Los Angeles Atherosclerosis Study," *Journal of Clinical Endocrinology & Metabolism*, vol 95, no. 9 (2010): 4432-4440.

Chapter 15 - Premature menopause - when the change comes early

1. Spencer, RP, "Cessation of reproduction: an analytic view of menopause," *Medical Hypotheses*, vol. 59(4) (2002): pp 406-410.
2. A. Hoek, J. Schoemaker and H. A. Drexhage, "Premature ovarian failure and ovarian autoimmunity," *Endocrine Reviews*, vol. 18(1) (1997): pp 107-134.
3. DeBruin, ML, Huisbrink, J., *et al*, "Treatment-related risk factors for premature menopause following Hodgkin lymphoma," *Blood*, vol. 111 (2008): pp 101-108.
4. Panzer, C, Wise, S, Fantini, G, *et al*, "Impact of oral contraceptives on sex hormone-binding globulin and androgen levels: a retrospective study in women with sexual dysfunction," *Journal of Sexual Medicine*, vol. 3 (2006): pp 104–113.
5. Langrish, JP, Mills, NL, Bath, LE, *et al*, "Cardiovascular effects of physiological and standard sex steroid replacement regimens in premature ovarian failure," *Hypertension*, vol. 53 (2009): pp 805-811.
6. Oparil, S, "Hormone therapy of premature ovarian failure: the case for 'natural' estrogen," *Hypertension*, vol. 53 (2009): pp 745-746.
7. Woad K, Watkins W, Prendergart D, *et al*, "The genetic basis of premature ovarian failure," *Australian and New Zealand Journal of Obstetrics and Gynecology*, vol. 46. no.3 (2006): pp 242-244.

Chapter 16 - The women's health initiative study

1. Writing Group for the Women's Health Initiative Investigators, "Risks and benefits of estrogen plus progestin in healthy postmenopausal women: principal results from the Women's Health Initiative randomized controlled trial," *Journal of the American Medical Association*, vol. 288 (2002): pp 321-333.
2. Writing Group for the Women's Health Initiative Investigators, "Effects of conjugated equine estrogen in postmenopausal women with hysterectomy," *Journal of the American Medical Association*, vol. 291 (2004): pp 1701-1712.

3. Hulley, SB and Grady, D, "The WHI estrogen-alone trial - do things look any better?," *Journal of the American Medical Association*, vol. 291(14) (2004): pp 1769-1771.

4. Harman, S, Brinton, E, Cedars, M, *et al.*, "KEEPS: the Kronos Early Estrogen Prevention Study," *Climacteric*, vol. 8 (2005): p 3.

5. Gaspard, U, "Prevention of coronary heart disease by early postmenopausal hormone therapy: new supporting data," *European Journal of Obstetrics & Gynecology and Reproductive Biology*, (Paris), vol. 37(4) (2008): pp 340-345.

6. Rossouw, JE, Prentice, RL, Manson, JE, *et al*, "Postmenopausal hormone therapy and risk of cardiovascular disease by age and years since menopause," *Journal of the American Medical Association*, vol. 297(13) (2007): pp 1465-1477.

7. Stefanick, ML, Anderson, GL, Margolis, KL, *et al*, for the WHI Investigators, "Effects of conjugated equine estrogens on breast cancer and mammography screening in postmenopausal women with hysterectomy," *Journal of the American Medical Association*, vol. 295 (2006): pp 1647-1657.

8. Rohan, TE, Negassa, A, Chlebowski, RT, *et al*, "Conjugated equine estrogen and risk of benign proliferative breast disease: a randomized controlled trial," *Journal of National Cancer Institute*, vol. 100(10) (2008): p 754.

9. Prentice, RL, Chlebowski, RT, Stefanick, ML, *et al*, "Conjugated equine estrogens and breast cancer risk in the Women's Health Initiative clinical trial and observational study," *American Journal of Epidemiology*, vol. 167(12) (2008): pp 1407-1415.

10. Prentice, RL, *et al*, "Benefits and risks of postmenopausal hormone therapy when it is initiated soon after menopause," *American Journal of Epidemiology*, vol. 170 (2009): p 12.

11. Banks, E and Canfell, K, "Invited commentary: hormone therapy risks and benefits - the Women's Health Initiative findings and the postmenopausal estrogen timing hypothesis," *American Journal of Epidemiology*, vol. 170 (2009): p 24.

12. Kuhl, H and Stevenson, J, "The effect of medroxyprogesterone acetate on estrogen-dependent risks and benefits - an attempt to interpret the Women's Health Initiative results," *Gynecological Endocrinology*, vol. 22(6) (2006): pp 303-317.

13. Cirillo, DJ, Wallace, RB, Rodabough, RJ, *et al*, "Effect of estrogen therapy on gallbladder disease," *Journal of the American Medical Association* vol. 293(3) (2005): pp 330-339.

14. Turgeon, JL, McDonnell, DP, Wise, KA, and Wise, PM, "Hormone therapy: physiological complexity belies therapeutic simplicity," *Science*, vol. 304 (2004): pp 1269-1273.

15. Endocrine Society Scientific Statement, "Postmenopausal hormone therapy," *Journal of Clinical Endocrinology and Metabolism*, vol. 95(07) Supplement 1 (2010): pp S1-S66.

Chapter 17 - The timing hypothesis and the case for natural hormone

1. Dubey, RK, Imthurn, B, Barton, M, "Vascular consequences of menopause and hormone therapy: importance of timing of treatment and type of estrogen," *Cardiovascular Research*, vol. 66 (2005): pp 295-306.

2. Manson, JE and Bassuk, SS, "Invited commentary: hormone therapy and risk of coronary heart disease - why renew the focus on the early years of menopause?," *American Journal of Epidemiology*, vol. 166 (2007): p 511.

3. Barrett-Connor, E, "Hormones and heart disease in women: The timing hypothesis," *American Journal of Epidemiology*, vol. 166 (2007): p 506.

4. Prentice, RL, *et al*, "Benefits and risks of postmenopausal hormone therapy when it is initiated soon after menopause," *American Journal of Epidemiology*, vol. 170 (2009): p 12.

5. Banks, E and Canfell, K, "Invited commentary: Hormone therapy risks and benefits - The Women's Health Initiative findings and the postmenopausal estrogen timing hypothesis," *American Journal of Epidemiology*, vol. 170 (2009): p 24.

6. Dubey, RK, Tofovic, SP and Jackson, EK, "Cardiovascular pharmacology of estradiol metabolites," *Journal of Pharmacology and Experimental Therapeutics*, vol. 308(2) (2004): pp 403-409.

7. Turgeon, JL, McDonnell, DP, Wise, KA, and Wise, PM, "Hormone therapy: physiological complexity belies therapeutic simplicity," *Science*, vol. 304 (2004): pp 1269-1273.

8. Bourghardt, J, Bergstrom, G, Krettek, A, *et al*, "The endogenous estradiol metabolite 2-methoxyestradiol reduces atherosclerotic lesion formation in female apolipoprotein E deficient mice," *Endocrinology*, vol. 148(9) (2007): pp 4128-4132.

9. Dubey, RK, Imthurn, B and Jackson, EK, "2-methoxyestradiol: a potential treatment for multiple proliferative disorders," *Endocrinology*, vol. 148(9) (2007): pp 4124-4127..

10. Mooberry, SL, "New insights into 2-methoxyestradiol, a promising antiangiogenic and antitumor agent," *Current Opinion in Oncology*, vol. 15 (2003): pp 425-430.

11. Dantas, APV and Sandberg, K, "Does 2-methoxyestradiol represent the new and improved hormone replacement therapy for atherosclerosis?," *Circulation Research*, vol. 99 (2006): pp 234-237.

12. Novensa L, Selent J, Pastor M, *et al*, "Equine estrogens impair nitric oxide production and endothelial nitric oxide synthase transcription in human endothelial cells compared with the natural 17-beta-estradiol." *Hypertension*, vol. 56 (2010): pp 405.

13. Barton M and Meyer MR, "Postmenopausal hypertension: Mechanisms and therapy," *Hypertension*, vol 54 (2009): pp 11-18.

14. Silverman DH, Geist CL, Kenna HA, *et al*, "Differences in regional brain metabolism associated with specific formulations of hormone therapy in postmenopausal women at risk for AD," *Psychoneuroendocrinology*, Aug. 30, 2010. (Epub ahead of print).

15. Tevaarwerk AJ, Holen KD Allberti DB, *et al*, "Phase I Trial of 2-methoxyestradiol Nano Crystal dispersion in advanced solid malignancies," *Clinical Cancer Research*, vol 15 (2009):pp 1460-1465.

16. Verenich S and Gerk PM, "Therapeutic promises of 2-methoxyestradiol and its drug disposition challenges," *Molecular Pharmaceutics*, DOI: 10.1021/mp100190f Publication Date (Web): September 10, 2010.

17. Toh S, Hernandez-Diaz S, Logan R, *et al*, "Coronary heart disease in postmenopausal recipients of estrogen plus progestin therapy: does the increased risk ever disappear?" *Annals of Internal Medicine*, vol. 152 (2010): pp 211-217.

18. Harman SSM, Brinton EA, Naftolin F, *et al*, "Comments on Toh article: Duration and timing effects on risks and benefits of menopausal hormones," *Annals of Internal Medicine*, published online March 10, 2010.

19. Pines A and Sturdee D, "Comments on Toh article: Discrepancy between authors' abstract and summary for women," *Annals of Internal Medicine*, published online March 29, 2010.

20. Toh S, Rossouw JE and Hernan MA, "Authors' response," *Annals of Internal Medicine*, published online April 7, 2010

Chapter 18 - Factors to consider before assessing risk of HRT

1. Hodis, HN and Mack, WJ, "Postmenopausal hormone therapy in clinical perspective", *Menopause*, vol. 13, no. 5 (2007): pp 944-957.

2. Hodis, HN, "Assessing benefits and risks of hormone therapy in 2008: new evidence, especially with regard to the heart," *Cleveland Clinic Journal of Medicine*, vol 75(4) (2008): pp S3-S12.

3. McKenzie, M, Sikon, AL, Thacker, HL, *et al*, "Putting the latest data into practice: case studies and clinical considerations in menopausal management," *Cleveland Clinic Journal of Medicine*, vol 75(4) (2008): pp S25-S33.

4. Schottenfeld D, Fraumeni JF Jr., Editors: Grady D, Ernster VL, "Endometrial cancer," *Cancer Epidemiology and Prevention*, 2nd Ed. New York (NY): Oxford University Press, (1996) pp. 1058-1089.

5. Weiderpass, E, Adami, HO, Baron, JA, *et al*, "Risk of endometrial cancer following estrogen replacement with and without progestins," *Journal of National Cancer Institute*, vol. 91 (1999): pp 1131-1137.

6. Archer, DF, "The effect of the duration of progestin use on the occurrence of endometrial cancer in postmenopausal women," *Menopause*, vol. 8, no. 4 (2001): pp 245-251.

7. Heron, M, Hoyert, DL, Murphy, SL, *et al*, "Deaths: final data for 2006," *National Vital Statistics Reports*, vol. 57, no. 14 (2009): pp 1-135.

8. Ford, ES, Bergmann, MM, Kroger, J, *et al*, "Healthy living is the best revenge," *Archives of Internal Medicine*, vol. 169, no.15 (2009): pp 1355-1362.

9. Rosner, B, Colditz, GA, Willet, WC, "Reproductive risk factors in a prospective study of breast cancer: the Nurses' Health Study," *American Journal of Epidemiology*, vol. 139, no. 8 (1994): pp 819-835.

10. Irwin, ML, Aiello, EJ, *et al*, "Physical activity, body mass index and mammographic density in postmenopausal breast cancer survivors," *Journal of Clinical Oncology*, vol. 25(9) (2007): pp 1061-1066.

11. Tamimi, RM, Byme, C, Colditz, GA, *et al*, "Endogenous hormone levels, mammographic density, and subsequent risk of breast cancer in postmenopausal women," *Journal of National Cancer Institute*, vol. 99, no. 15 (2007): pp 1178-1187.

12. Kaaks, R, Rinaldi, S, Key, TJ, *et al*, "Postmenopausal serum androgens, oestrogens, and breast cancer risk: the European prospective investigation into cancer and nutrition," *Endocrine-Related Cancer*, vol. 12 (2005): pp 1071-1082.

13. Boyd, NF, Greenberg, C, *et al*, "Effects at two years of a low-fat high-carbohydrate diet on radiologic features of the breast: results from a randomized trial," Canadian Diet and Breast Cancer Prevention Study Group, *Journal of National Cancer Institute*, vol. 89(7) (1997): pp 488-96.

14. Feigelson, HS, Jonas, CR, *et al*, "Weight gain, body mass index, hormone replacement therapy, and postmenopausal breast cancer in a large prospective study," *Cancer Epidemiology, Biomarkers, and Prevention*, vol. 13 (2004): p 220.

15. Eliassen, AH, Colditz, GA, *et al*, "Adult weight change and risk of postmenopausal breast cancer," *Journal of the American Medical Association*, vol. 296(2) (2006): pp 193-201.

16. *American Cancer Society*: Breast Cancer Facts and Figures, 2007-2008. Atlanta: American Cancer Society, Inc.

17. Allen, N, *et al*, "Moderate alcohol intake and cancer incidence in women," *Journal of National Cancer Institute*, vol. 101 (2009): pp 296-305.

18. Lauer, M. and Sorlie, P., "Alcohol, cardiovascular disease and cancer: treat with caution," *Journal of National Cancer Institute*, vol. 101(2009): pp 282-283.

19. Collaborative Group on Hormonal Factors in Breast Cancer, "Breast cancer and breast feeding: collaborative reanalysis of individual data from 47 epidemiological studies in 30 countries, including 50302 women with breast cancer and 96973 women without the disease," *The Lancet*, vol. 360, no. 9328 (2002): pp 187-195.

20. Hartmann, LC, Sellers, TA, *et al*, "Benign breast disease and risk of breast cancer," *New England Journal of Medicine*, vol. 353, no. 3 (2005): pp 229-237.

21. Gateley, CA, Maddox, PR, Mansel, RE, *et al*, "Mastalgia refractory to drug treatment," *British Journal of Surgery*, vol. 77 (1990): pp 1110.

22. Gateley, CA, Maddox, PR, Pritchard, GA, *et al*, "Plasma fatty acid profiles in benign breast disorders," *British Journal of Surgery*, vol. 79 (1992): p 407.

23. London RS, Murphy L, Kitlowski KE, *et al*, "Efficacy of alpha-tocopherol in the treatment of the premenstrual syndrome," *The Journal of Reproductive Medicine*, vol. 32 (1987): p 400.

24. Yin, L, Grandi, N, Raum, E, *et al*, "Meta-analysis: serum vitamin D and breast cancer risk," *European Journal of Cancer*, vol. 46, no. 12 (2010): pp 2196-2205.

25. Chen, P, Pingting H, Dong X, *et al*, (June 2010), Meta-analysis of vitamin D, calcium, and the prevention of breast cancer, *Breast Cancer Research and Treatment*, vol. 121, no. 2 (2010): pp 469-477.

26. Krishnan, AV, Swami, S and Feldman, D, "Vitamin D and breast cancer: inhibition of estrogen synthesis and signaling," *The Journal of Steroid Biochemistry and Molecular Biology*, vol. 121, no. 1-2 (2010): pp 343-348.

27. Kabat, GC, O'Leary, ES, Gammon, MD, *et al*, "Estrogen metabolism and breast cancer," *Epidemiology*, vol. 17 (2006): pp 80-88.

28. Jernstrom, H, Klug, TL, *et al*, "Predictors of the plasma ratio of 2-hydroxyestrone to 16-alpha hydroxyestrone among premenopausal, nulliparous women from four ethnic groups," *Carcinogenesis*, vol. 24 no. 5 (2003): pp 991-1005.

29. Bradlow, HL, Jernstrom, H, *et al*, "Comparison of plasma and urinary levels of 2-hydroxyestrogen and 16-alpha hydroxyestrogen metabolites," *Molecular Genetics and Metabolism*, vol. 87 (2005): pp 135-146.

30. Miller, K, "Estrogen and DNA damage: the silent source of breast cancer?," *Journal of National Cancer Institute*, vol. 95, no. 2 (2003): pp 100-102.

31. Yager JD and Davidson NE, "Estrogen carcinogenesis in breast cancer," *New England Journal of Medicine*, vol. 354 (2006): pp 270-282.

32. Cummings, SR, Tice, JA, Bauer, S, "Prevention of breast cancer in postmenopausal women: approaches to estimating and reducing risk," *Journal of National Cancer Institute*, vol. 101 (2009): pp 384-398.

33. Yue, W, Santen, RJ, Wang, JP, Rogan, EG, *et al*, "Genotoxic metabolites of estradiol in breast: potential mechanism of estradiol induced carcinogenesis," *The Journal of Steroid Biochemistry and Molecular Biology*, vol. 86, no. 3-5 (2003): pp 477-486.

34. Cavalieri, E, Chakravarti, D, Guttenplan, J, Rogan, E, *et al*, "Catechol estrogen quinones as initiators of breast and other human cancers: implications for biomarkers of susceptibility and cancer prevention," *Biochimica et Biophysica Acta*, vol. 1766, no. 1 (2006): pp 63-78.

35. Cavalleri, EL and Rogan, EG, "A unifying mechanism in the initiation of cancer and other diseases by catechol quinones," *Annals of New York Academy of Science*, vol. 1028 (2004): pp 247-257.

36. Yue, W, Wang, JP, Li, Y, Rogan, E, *et al*, "Tamoxifen versus aromatase inhibitors for breast cancer prevention," *Clinical Cancer Research*, vol. 11, no. 2, pt. 2 (2005): pp 925s-930s.

37. Napoli, N, Donepudi, S, *et al*, "Increased 2-hydroxylation of estrogen in women with a family history of osteoporosis," *The Journal of Clinical Endocrinology and Metabolism*, vol. 90, no. 4 (2005): pp 2035-2041.

38. Dubey, RK, Gillespie, DG, Zacharia, LC, *et al*, "Methoxyestradiols mediate the antimitogenic effects of estradiol on vascular smooth muscle cells via estrogen receptor-independent mechanisms," *Biochemical and Biophysical Research Communication*, vol. 278 (2000): pp 27–33.

39. Zacharia, LC, Jackson, EK, Gillespie, DG, Dubey, RK, "Catecholamines abrogate the antimitogenic effects of 2-hydroxyestradiol on human aortic vascular smooth muscle cells," *Arteriosclerosis, Thrombosis, and Vascular Biology*, vol. 21 (2001): pp 1745-1750.

40. Zacharia, LC, Jackson, EK, DG, Dubey, RK, "Increased 2-methoxyestradiol production in human coronary versus aortic vascular cells.," *Hypertension*, vol. 37, pt. 2 (2001): pp 658 – 662.

41. Dubey, RK, Gillespie, DG, *et al*, "Methoxyestradiols mediate the antimitogenic effects of locally applied estradiol on cardiac fibroblast growth," *Hypertension*, vol. 39 (2002): pp 412– 417.

42. Brooks, JD, Ward, WE, *et al*, "Supplementation with flaxseed alters estrogen metabolism in postmenopausal women to a greater extent than does supplementation with an equal amount of soy," *American Journal of Clinical Nutrition*, vol. 79 (2004): pp 318-325.

43. Verschraegen C, Vinh-Hung V, Cserni G, *et al*, "Modeling the effect of tumor size in early breast cancer," *Annals of Surgery*, vol. 241, no. 2 (2005): pp 309-315.
    US Preventive Services Task Force, "Screening for breast cancer: US Preventive Services Task Force recommendation statement," *Annals of Internal Medicine*, vol. 151, no.10 (2009): pp 716-726.

44. Heliquist, B, Duffy, S, Absaleh, S, *et al*, "Effectiveness of population-based service screening with mammography for women ages 40-49," *Cancer* (2010): DOI:10.1002/cncr.25650.

45. US Preventive Services Task Force, "Risk assessment and BRCA mutation testing for breast and ovarian cancer susceptibility: recommendation statement," *Annals of Internal Medicine*, vol. 143 (2005): pp 355-361.

46. Afonso, N, "Women at high risk for breast cancer - what the primary care provider needs to know," *The Journal of the American Board of Family Medicine*, vol. 22 (2009): pp 43-50.

47. Foster, RS, Lang, SP, and Costanza, MC, "Breast self-examination practices and breast cancer stage," *New England Journal of Medicine*, vol. 299 (1978): pp 265-270.

48. Saslow, D, Hannah, J, Osuch, J, Pennypacker, H, *et al*, "Clinical breast examination: practical recommendations for optimizing performance and reporting," *CA: A Cancer Journal for Clinicians*, vol. 54, no. 6 (2004): pp 327-344.

49. Pennypacker, HS, Naylor, L, Sander, AA and Goldstein, MK, "Why can't we do better breast examinations?," *Nurse Practitioner Forum*, vol. 10, no. 3 (1999): pp 122-128.

Chapter 19 - Risks from any hormone replacement therapy

1. Collaborative Group on Hormonal Factors in Breast Cancer, "Breast cancer and hormone replacement therapy: collaborative reanalysis of data from 51 epidemiological studies of 52,705 women with breast cancer and 108,411 women without breast cancer," *The Lancet*, vol. 350 (1997): p 1047-1059.

2. Ries, LAG, Harkins, D, Krapcho, M, *et al*, "SEER cancer statistics review, 1975-2003," Bethesda, MD; *National Cancer Institute* (2006).

3. Collins, JA, Blake, JM and Crosignani, PG, "Breast cancer risk with postmenopausal hormone treatment," *Human Reproductive Update*, vol. 11 (2005): pp 545-560.

4. Stefanick, ML, Anderson, GL, Margolis, KL, *et al*, "Effects of conjugated equine estrogens on breast cancer and mammography screening in postmenopausal women with hysterectomy," *Journal of the American Medical Association*, vol. 295, no. 14 (2006): pp 1647-1657.

5. Fournier, A, Mesrinne, S, Boutron-Ruault, *et al*, "Estrogen progestogen menopausal hormone therapy and breast cancer: does delay from menopause onset to treatment initiation influence risks?," *Journal of Clinical Oncology*, vol. 27 (2009): pp 5138-5143.

6. Bernstein, L, Editorial. "Combined hormone therapy at menopause and breast cancer: a warning - short-term use increases risk," *Journal of Clinical Oncology*, vol. 27 (2009): pp 5116-5119.

7. Stoll, BA, "Hypothesis: breast cancer regression under oestrogen therapy," *British Medical Journal*, vol. J 3 (1973): pp 446-450.

8. Ingle, JN, *et al*, "Randomized clinical trial of diethylstilbesterol versus tamoxifen in postmenopausal women with advanced breast cancer," *New England Journal of Medicine*, vol. 304 (1981): pp 16-21.

9. Ellis, MJ, *et al*, "Lower-dose vs high-dose oral estradiol therapy of hormone receptor-positive aromatase inhibitor-resistant advanced breast cancer: Al phase 2 randomized study," *Journal of the American Medical Association*, vol. 302 (2009): pp 774-780.

10. Munster, PN and Carpenter, JT, "Estradiol in breast cancer treatment: reviving the past," *Journal of the American Medical Association*, vol. 302 (2009): pp 797-798.

11. Mack, TM, Pike, MC, *et al*, "Estrogens and endometrial cancer in a retirement community," *New England Journal of Medicine*, vol. 294 (1976): pp 1262-1267.

12. Renehan, AG, Tyson, M, *et al*, "Body mass index and incidence of cancer: a systematic review and meta-analysis of prospective observational studies," *The Lancet*, vol. 371, no. 9612 (2008): pp 569-578.

13. Calle EE, Rodriguqz D, *et al*, "Overweight, obesity, and mortality from cancer in a prospectively studied cohort of US adults," *New England Journal of Medicine*, vol. 348 (2003): pp 1625-1638.

14. Reeves, GK, Pirie, K, *et al*, "Cancer incidence and mortality in relation to body mass index in the Million Women Study: cohort study," *British Medical Journal*, vol. 335 (2007) : pp 1134-1139.

15. Barratt, A, Wyer, PC, Hatala, R, *et al*, "Tips for learners of evidence-based medicine: 1. relative risk reduction, absolute risk reduction, and number needed to treat," *Canadian Medical Association Journal*, vol. 171, no. 4 (2004): pp 353-358.

16. Grady, D, Gebretsadik, T, *et al*, "Hormone replacement therapy and endometrial cancer risk: a meta-analysis," *Obstetrics and Gynecology*, vol. 85 (1995): pp 304-313.

17. Thomas, CC, *et al*, "Endometrial cancer risk among younger, overweight women," *Obstetrics and Gynecology*, vol. 114 (2009): p 22.

18. Weiderpass, Elisabete, Adami, Hans-Olov, *et al*, "Risk of endometrial cancer following estrogen replacement with and without progestins," *Journal of National Cancer Institute*, vol. 171, no. 4 (2004): pp 353-358.

19. Lacey, JV Jr., Leitzmann, MF, Chang, SC, *et al*, "Endometrial cancer and menopausal hormone therapy in the National Institutes of Health-AARP Diet and Health Study cohort," *Cancer*, vol. 109, no. 7 (2007): pp 1303-1311.

20. Archer, DF, "The effect of the duration of progestin use on the occurrence of endometrial cancer in postmenopausal women," *Menopause*, vol. 8, no. 4 (2001): pp 245-251.

21. Rossouw, JE, Anderson, GI, Prentice, RL, *et al*, "Risks and benefits of estrogen plus progestin in healthy postmenopausal women: principal results from the Women's Health Initiative randomized controlled trial," *Journal of the American Medical Association*, vol. 288, no. 3 (2002): pp 321-333.

22. *The National Heart Lung and Blood Institute*, "Postmenopausal hormone therapy: facts about postmenopausal hormone therapy," www.nhlbi.nih.gov/health/women/pht_facts.htm. Accessed June 28, 2005.

23. Weiss, LK, Burkman, RT, *et al*, "Hormone replacement therapy regimens and breast cancer risk," *Obstetrics and Gynecology*, vol. 100, no. 6 (2002): pp 1148-1158.

24. National Council on Aging, "Myths and perceptions about aging and women's health, assessing the odds," *The Lancet*, vol. 350, no. 9091 (1997): p 1563.

25. Black, WC, Nease, RF, and Tosteson, AN, "Perceptions of breast cancer risk and screening effectiveness in women younger than 50 years of age," *Journal of National Cancer Institute*, vol. 87, no. 10 (1995): pp 720-731.

26. Harman, SM, "Estrogen replacement in menopausal women: recent and current prospective studies, the WHI and the KEEPS," *Gender Medicine*, vol. 3, no. 4 (2006): pp 254-269.

27. Fournier, A, Berrino, F, and Clavel-Chapelon, F, "Unequal risks for breast cancer associated with different hormone replacement therapies: results from the E3N cohort study," *Breast Cancer Research and Treatment*, vol 107, no. 1 (2008): pp 1033-1111.

28. Chlebowski, R, *et al*, "Breast cancer risk declines quickly after stopping hormone therapy," *New England Journal of Medicine*, vol. 360 (2009): pp 573-587.

29. Beral, V, *et al*, "Ovarian cancer and hormone replacement therapy in the Million Women Study," *The Lancet*, vol. 369, no. 9574 (2007): pp 1703-1710.

30. Canonico, M, Plu-Bureau, G, *et al*, "Hormone replacement therapy and risk of venous thromboembolism in postmenopausal women: systematic review and meta-analysis," *British Medical Journal*, vol. 336 (2008): pp 1227-1231.

31. de Lignieres, B, de Vathaire, F., *et al*, "Combined hormone replacement therapy and risk of breast cancer in a French cohort study of 3175 women," *Climacteric*, vol. 5, no. 4 (2002): pp 332-340.

32. Position Statement, "Estrogen and progestogen use in postmenopausal women: position statement of The North American Menopause Society," *Menopause*, vol. 15, no. 4 (2008): pp 584-602.

33. Million Women Study Collaborators, "Breast cancer and hormone-replacement therapy in the Million Women Study," *The Lancet*, vol. 362, no. 9382 (2003): pp 419-427.

34. Rohan TE, Negassa, A, Chlebowski, RT, *et al*, "Conjugated equine estrogen and risk of benign proliferative breast disease: a randomized controlled trial," *Journal of National Cancer Institute*, vol. 100, no. 8 (2008): pp 563-571.

35. Schaumberg, DA, Buring, JE, Sullivan, DA, Dana, MR, "Hormone replacement therapy and dry eye syndrome," *Journal of the American Medical Association,* vol. 286 (2001): p 2114.

36. Fraenkel, Y, Chaisson, CE, Evans, SR, *et al,* "The association of estrogen replacement therapy and the Raynaud phenomenon in postmenopausal women," *Annals of Internal Medicine,* vol. 129, no. 3 (1998): pp 208-211.

37. Hepburn, MJ, Dooley, DP, Morris, MJ, "The effects of estrogen replacement therapy on airway function in postmenopausal, asthmatic women," *Archives of Internal Medicine,* vol. 161, no. 22 (2001): pp 2717-2720.

38. Lieberman, D, Kopernik, G, *et al,* "Sub-clinical worsening of bronchial asthma during estrogen replacement therapy in asthmatic post-menopausal women," *Maturitas,* vol. 21, no. 2 (1995): pp 153-157.

39. Troisi, RJ, Speizer, FE, *et al,* "Menopause, postmenopausal estrogen preparations, and the risk of adult-onset asthma: a prospective cohort study," *American Journal of Respiratory and Critical Care Medicine,* vol. 152, no. 4, pt. 1 (1995): pp 1183-1188.

40. Harden, CL, Pulver, MC, *et al,* "The effect of menopause and perimenopause on the course of epilepsy," *Epilepsia,* vol. 40, no. 10 (1999): pp 1402-1407.

41. Urowitz, MB, Ibanez, D, Jerome, D, Gladman, DD, "The effect of menopause on disease activity in systemic lupus erythematosus," *The Journal of Rheumatology,* vol. 33, no. 11 (2006): pp 2192-2198.

42. Sanchez-Guerrero, J, Liang, MH, *et al,* "Postmenopausal estrogen therapy and the risk for developing systemic lupus erythematosus," *Annals of Internal Medicine,* vol. 122, no. 6 (1995): pp 430-433.

43. Ang, WC, Farrell, E, Vollenhoven, B, "Effect of hormone replacement therapies and selective estrogen receptor modulators in postmenopausal women with uterine leiomyomas: a literature review," *Climacteric,* vol. 4, no. 4 (2001): pp 284-292.

44. Yang, CH; Lee, JN; Hsu, SC, "Effect of hormone replacement therapy on uterine fibroids in postmenopausal women - a 3-year study," *Maturitas*, vol. 43, no. 1 (2002): pp 35-39.

45. Ascherio, A, Chen, H, Schwarzschiled, MA, *et al*, "Caffeine, postmenopausal estrogen, and risk of Parkinson's disease," *Neurology*, vol. 60, no. 5 (2003): pp 790-795.

46. *Radiological Society of North America* (RSNA) 95th Scientific Assembly and Annual Meeting: Abstract RO22-04. Presented November 30, 2009.

Chapter 20 - Increased risks from oral estrogens

1. Cirillo, DJ, Wallace, RB, and Rodabough, RJ, "Effect of estrogen therapy on gallbladder disease," *Journal of the American Medical Association*, vol. 295 (2005): pp 330-339.

2. Uhler, ML, Marks, JW, Voigt, BJ, and Judd, HL, "Comparison of the impact of transdermal versus oral estrogen on biliary markers of gallstone formation in postmenopausal women," *Journal of Clinical Endocrinology and Metabolism*, vol. 83, no. 2 (1998): pp 410-414.

3. Liu, B, Beral, V, Balkwill, A, *et al*, "Gallbladder disease and use of transdermal versus oral hormone replacement therapy in postmenopausal women: prospective cohort study," *British Medical Journal*, vol. 337 (2008): p a386.

4. AACE Menopause Guidelines Revision Task Force, "American Association of Clinical Endocrinologists medical guidelines for clinical practice for the diagnosis and treatment of menopause," *Endocrine Practice*, vol. 12 (2006): pp 315-337.

5. Sare, GM, Gray, LJ and Bath, PMW, "Association between hormone replacement therapy and subsequent arterial and venous vascular events: a meta-analysis," *European Heart Journal*, vol. 29 (2008): pp 2031-2041.

6. Vongpatanasin, W, Tuncel, M, Mansour, Y, Arbique, D, Victor, RG, "Transdermal estrogen replacement therapy decreases sympathetic activity in postmenopausal women," *Circulation*, vol. 103 (2001): pp 2903-2908.

7.   Scarabin, PY, Oger, E, Plu-Bureau, G; "Estrogen and thromboembolism risk study group. Differential association of oral and transdermal oestrogen-replacement therapy with venous thromboembolism risk," *The Lancet*, vol. 362 (2003): pp 428-432.

8.   Herrington, DM and Parks, JS, "Estrogen and HDL, all that glitters is not gold, arteriosclerosis, thrombosis and vascular biology", *Arteriosclerosis, Thrombosis and Vascular Biology*, vol. 24 (2004): pp 1741-1742.

9.   Shifren, JL, "A comparison of the short-term effects of oral conjugated equine estrogens versus transdermal estradiol on C-reactive protein, other serum markers of inflammation, and other hepatic proteins in naturally menopausal women," *Journal of Clinical Endocrinology and Metabolism*, vol. 93, no. 5 (2008): pp 1702-1710.

10. Shrifrin, JL, Desindes, S, McIlwain, M, Doros, G, Mazer, NA, "A randomized, open-label crossover study comparing the effects of oral versus transdermal estrogen therapy on serum androgens, thyroid hormones, and adrenal hormones in naturally menopausal women," *Menopause*, vol. 14 (2007): pp 985-994.

11. Straczek, C, Oger, E, Yon de Jonage-Canonico, MB, *et al*, "Prothrombothic mutations, hormone therapy, and venous thromboembolism among postmenopausal women: impact of the route of estrogen administration," *Circulation*, vol. 112 (2005): pp 3495-3500.

12. Abbas, A, Fadel, P, Wang, Z, *et al*, "Contrasting effects of oral versus transdermal estrogen on serum amyloid A (SAA) and high-density lipoprotein-SAA in postmenopausal women,"*Arteriosclerosis, Thrombosis, and Vascular Biology*, vol. 24 (2004): pp e164-e167.

13. O'Connell, MB, "Pharmacokinetic and pharmacologic variation between different estrogen products," *The Journal of Clinical Pharmacology*, vol. 35 (suppl) (1995): pp 18S-24S.

14. Walsh, BW, Schiff, I, Rosner, B, *et al*, "Effects of postmenopausal estrogen replacement on the concentrations and metabolism of plasma lipoproteins," *New England Journal of Medicine*, vol. 325, no. 17 (1991): pp 1196-1204.

15. Darling, GM, Johns, JA and McCloud, PI, *et al*, "Estrogen and progestin compared with simvastatin for hypercholesterolemia in postmenopausal women," *New England Journal of Medicine*, vol. 337, no. 9 (1997): pp 595-601.

16. Hanington E, Jones R, Amess J, "Platelet aggregation in response to 5HT in migraine patients taking oral contraceptives," *The Lancet*, vol. 1 (1982): pp 967-968.

17. Goodman, MP, "Is there any role for oral estrogen therapy? The Case for Transdermal Therapy as of 2009?", Abstract Presented at the 20th Annual Meeting of the North America Menopause Society, San Diego, California. (2009).

18. Colao A, Spiezia S, *et al*, "Circulating insulin-like growth factor-1 levels are correlated with the atherosclerotic profile in healthy subjects independently of age," *Journal of Endocrinology Investigation*, vol. 28 (2005): pp 440-448.

19. Slater CC, Hodis HN, Mack WJ, *et al*, "Markedly elevated levels of estrone sulfate after long-term oral, but not transdermal, administration of estradiol in postmenopausal women," *Menopause*, vol. 8 (2001): pp 200-203.

20. Johnson SP, Hundborg HH, *et al*, "Insulin-like growth factor (IGF-1) I-II and IGF binding protein-3 and risk of ischemic stroke," *Journal of Clinical Endocrinology and Metabolism*, vol. 90 (2005): pp 5937-5941.

21. Nachtigall LE, Raju U, Banerjee S, *et al*, "Serum estradiol-binding profiles in postmenopausal women undergoing three common estrogen replacement therapies: associations with sex hormone binding globulin, estradiol, and estrone levels," *Menopause*, vol. 7 (2000): pp 243-250.

22. DeCarlo C, Tommaselli G, *et al*, "Serum leptin levels and body composition in postmenopausal women: effects of hormone therapy," *Menopause*, vol. 11, no. 4 (2004): pp 466-473.

23. Lwin R, Darnell B, Oster R, *et al*, "Effect of oral estrogen on substrate utilization in postmenopausal women," *Fertility and Sterility*, vol. 90, no. 4 (2008): pp 1275-1278.

24. O'Sullivan AJ, Crampton LJ, Freund, *et al*, "The route of estrogen replacement therapy confers divergent effects on substrate oxidation and body composition in postmenopausal women," *The Journal of Clinical Investigation*, vol. 102 (1998): pp 1035-1040.

25. Chu MC, Cosper P and Lobo RA, "Comparison of oral and transdermal estradiol therapy on insulin resistance parameters in postmenopausal women," *Fertility and Sterility*, vol. 84 (supp 1) (2005): p S121.

26. Chu MC, Cushman M, Solomon R, *et al*, "Metabolic syndrome in postmenopausal women: the influence of oral or transdermal estradiol on inflammation and coagulation markers," *American Journal of Obstetrics and Gynecology*, vol. 199 (2008): pp 526.e1-526.e7.

27. Chu MC, Cosper P, Nakhuda GS, *et al*, "A comparison of oral and transdermal short-term estrogen therapy in postmenopausal women with metabolic syndrome," *Fertility and Sterility*, vol. 86 no. 6 (2006): pp 1669-1675.

28. Shifren J, Desindes S, MD, *et al*, "A randomized, open-label, crossover study comparing the effects of oral versus transdermal estrogen therapy on serum androgens, thyroid hormones, and adrenal hormones in naturally menopausal women," *Menopause*, vol. 14, no. 6 (2007): pp 985-994.

29. Nappi RE, Polatti F, "The use of estrogen therapy in women's sexual functioning," *Journal of Sexual Medicine*, vol. 6, no. 3 (2009): pp 603-616.

30. Ropponen A, Aittomaki K, Vihma V, *et al*, "Effects of oral and transdermal estradiol administration on levels of sex hormone-binding globulin in postmenopausal women with and without a history of intrahepatic cholestatis of pregnancy," *Journal of Clinical Endocrinology and Metabolism*, vol. 90, no. 6 (2005): pp 3431-3434.

31. Vehkavaara S, Hakala-Ala-Pietila T, Virkamaki A, *et al*, "Differential effects of oral and transdermal estrogen replacement therapy on endothelial function in postmenopausal women," *Circulation*, vol. 102 (2000): pp 2687-2693.

32. Modena MG, Bursi F, Fantini G, *et al*, "Effects of hormone replacement therapy on c-reactive protein levels in healthy postmenopausal women: comparison between oral and transdermal administration of estrogen," *American Journal of Medicine*, vol. 113 (2002): pp 331-334.

33. Modena MG, Sismondi P, *et al*, "New evidence regarding hormone replacement therapies is urgently required transdermal postmenopausal hormone therapy differs from oral hormone therapy in risks and benefits," *Maturitas*, vol. 52, no. 1 (2005): pp 1-10.

34. Martin VT, Behbehani M, "Ovarian hormones and migraine headache: understanding mechanisms and pathogenesis," *Headache*, vol. 46, no. 3 (2006): pp 365-386.

35. Vehkavaara S, Silveira A, Hakala-ala-Pietila T, *et al*, "Effects of oral and transdermal estrogen replacement therapy on markers of coagulation, fibrinolysis, inflammation and serum lipids and lipoproteins in postmenopausal women," *Journal of Thrombosis and Haemostasis*, vol. 85 (2001): pp 619-625.

36. Boostanfar RS, Saada T, Poysky J, *et al*, "Serum endocrine markers and psychosocial mood in postmenopausal women: The difference between transdermal and oral HRT," Presented at: 10th World Congress on Menopause; Berlin, Germany (June 2002).

37. L'Hermite ML, Simoncini T, Fuller S, *et al*, "Could transdermal estradiol + progesterone be a safer postmenopausal HRT? A Review," *Maturitas*, vol. 60 (2002): pp 185-201.

38. Clendenen TV, Koenig KL, Shore RE, *et al*, "Postmenopausal levels of endogenous sex hormones and risk of colorectal cancer," *Cancer Epidemiology, Biomarkers & Prevention*, vol. 18, no. 1 (2009): pp 275-281.

Chapter 21 - Increased risks of adding daily oral progestin to oral estrogens

1. Ottosson UB, Johansson BG, von Schoultz B, (1985 Mar 15) "Subfractions of high-density lipoprotein cholesterol during estrogen replacement therapy: a comparison between progestogens and natural progesterone," *American Journal of Obstetrics and Gynecology*, vol. 151, no. 6 (1985): pp 746-750.

2. Moorjani S; Dupont A; Labrie F, *et al*, (1991 Aug) "Changes in plasma lipoprotein and apolipoprotein composition in relation to oral versus percutaneous administration of estrogen alone or in cyclic association with utrogestan in menopausal women", *Journal of Clinical Endocrinology and Metabolism*, vol. 73, no. 2 (1991): pp 373-379.

3. Renoux C, Dell Aniello S, Garbe E, *et al*, "Transdermal and oral hormone replacement therapy and the risk of stroke: a nested case-control study," *British Medical Journal*, vol. 340 (2010): pp c2519.

4. Hulley SB, Grady D, "The WHI estrogen-alone trial - do things look any better?," *Journal of the American Medical Association*, vol. 291, no. 14 (2004): pp 1769-1771.

5. Writing Group for the Women's Health Initiative Investigators, "Effects of conjugated equine estrogen in postmenopausal women with hysterectomy," *Journal of the American Medical Association*, vol. 291 (2004): pp 1701-1712.

6. Writing Group for the Women's Health Initiative Investigators, "Risks and benefits of estrogen plus progestin in healthy postmenopausal women: principal results from the Women's Health Initiative randomized controlled trial," *Journal of the American Medical Association*, vol. 288 (2002): pp 321-333.

7. Li CI, Malone KE, Porter PL, *et al*, "Relationship between long durations and different regimens of hormone therapy and risk of breast cancer," *Journal of the American Medical Association*, vol. 289, no. 24 (2003): pp 3254-3263.

8. Ory K, Lebeau L, Levalois C, *et al*, "Apoptosis inhibition mediated by medroxyprogesterone acetate treatment of breast cancer ce," *Breast Cancer Research and Treatment*, vol. 68 (2001): pp 187-198.

9. Eigeliene N, Harkonen P, Erkkola R, "Effects of estradiol and medroxyprogesterone acetate on morphology, proliferation and apoptosis of human breast tissue in organ cultures," *BioMed Central Cancer*, vol. 6 (2006): pp 246.

10. Schramek D, Leibbrandt A, Sigl V, *et al*, "Osteoclast differentiation factor RANK controls development of progestin-driven mammary cancer," *Nature*, published online 9/29/10 doi:10.1038/nature09387.

11. Beral V, "Breast cancer and hormone-replacement therapy in the Million Women Study," *The Lancet*, vol. 362, no. 9382 (2003): pp 419-427.

12. Tjonneland A, Christensen J, Thomsen B, *et al*, "Hormone replacement therapy in relation to breast carcinoma incidence rate ratios: a prospective Danish cohort study," *Cancer*, vol. 100, no. 11 (2004): pp 2328-2337.

13. Schairer C, Lubin J, Troisi R, *et al*, "Menopausal estrogen and estrogen-progestin replacement therapy and breast cancer risk," *Journal of the American Medical Association*, vol. 283, no. 4 (2000): pp 485-491.

14. Ross RK, Paganini-Hill A, Wan PC, *et al*, "Effect of hormone replacement therapy on breast cancer risk: estrogen versus estrogen plus progestin." *Journal of National Cancer Institute*, vol. 92, no. 4 (2000): pp 328-332.

15. Olsson HL, Ingvar C, Bladstrom A (2003 Mar 15) "Hormone replacement therapy containing progestins and given continuously increases breast carcinoma risk in Sweden," *Cancer*, vol. 97(6):pp 1387-1392.

16. Stahlberg C, Pedersen AT, Lynge E, *et al*, "Increased risk of breast cancer following different regimens of hormone replacement therapy frequently used in Europe," *International Journal of Cancer*, vol. 109, no. 5 (2004): pp 721-727.

17. Fournier A, Berrino F, Riboli E, *et al*, "Breast cancer risk in relation to different types of hormone replacement therapy in the E3N-EPIC cohort," *International Journal of Cancer*, vol. 114, no. 3 (2005): pp 448-454.

18. Chlebowski R, "Presentation to American Society of Clinical Oncology, 45th Annual Meeting," (2009).

19. Schabath MB, Wu X, Vassilopoulou-Sellin, *et al*, "Hormone replacement therapy and lung cancer risk: a case-control analysis," *Clinical Cancer Research*, vol. 10, no. 1, pt. 1 (2004): pp 113-123.

20. Blackman JA, Coogan PF, Rosenberg L, *et al*, "Estrogen replacement therapy and risk of lung cancer," *Pharmacoepidemiology and Drug Safety*, vol. 11, no. 7 (2002): pp 561-567.

21. Kreuzer M, Gerken M, Heinrich, *et al*, "Hormonal factors and risk of lung cancer among women?," *International Journal of Epidemiology*, vol. 32, no. 2 (2003): pp 263-271.

22. Chen KY, Hsiao CF, Chang GC, *et al*, "Hormone replacement therapy and lung cancer risk in Chinese," *Cancer*, vol. 110, no. 8 (2007): pp 1768-1775.

23. Schwartz AG, Wenzlaff AS, Prysak GM, *et al*, "Reproductive factors, hormone use, estrogen receptor expression and risk of non small-cell lung cancer in women," *Journal of Clinical Oncology*, vol. 25, no. 36 (2007): pp 5785-5792.

24. Rodriguez C, Feigelson HS, Deka A, *et al*, "Postmenopausal hormone therapy and lung cancer risk in the cancer prevention study II nutrition cohort," *Cancer Epidemiology, Biomarkers, and Prevention*, vol. 17, no. 3 (2008): pp 655-660.

25. Ayeni O, Robinson A, "Hormone replacement therapy and outcomes for women with non small cell lung cancer: can an association be confirmed?", *Current Oncology*, vol. 16, no. 3 (2009): pp 21-25.

26. Ganti AK, Sahmoun AE, Panwalkar AW, *et al*, "Hormone replacement therapy is associated with decreased survival in women with lung cancer," *Journal of Clinical Oncology*, vol. 24, no. 1 (2006): pp 59-63.

27. Ishibashi H, Suzuki T, Suzuke S, *et al*, "Progesterone receptor in non-small cell lung cancer: A potent prognostic factor and possible target for endocrine therapy," *Cancer Research*, vol. 65 (2005): pp 6450-6458.

28. Siegfried JM, "Hormone replacement therapy and decreased lung cancer survival," *Journal of Clinical Oncology*, vol. 24 (2006), p 9.

29. Matthews K, Cauley J, Yaffe K, *et al*, "Estrogen replacement therapy and cognitive decline in older community women," *Journal of the American Geriatrics Society*, vol. 47, no. 5 (1999): pp 518-523.

30. Kang JH, Weuve J, Grodstein F, "Postmenopausal hormone therapy and risk of cognitive decline in community-dwelling aging women," *Neurology*, vol. 63, no. 1 (2004): pp 101-107.

31. Rice MM, Graves AB, McCurry SM, *et al*, "Postmenopausal estrogen and estrogen-progestin use and 2-year rate of cognitive change in a cohort of older Japanese American women: The Kame Project," *Archives of Internal Medicine*, vol. 160, no. 11 (2000): pp 1641-1649.

32. Carlson MC, Zandi PP, Plassman BL, *et al*, "Hormone replacement therapy and reduced cognitive decline in older women: the Cache County Study," *Neurology*, vol. 57, no. 12 (2001) : pp 2210-2216.

33. Rapp SR, Espeland MA, Shumaker SA, *et al*, "Effect of estrogen plus progestin on global cognitive function in postmenopausal women: the Women's Health Initiative Memory Study: a randomized controlled trial," *Journal of the American Medical Association*, vol. 289, no. 20 (2003): pp 2663-2672.

34. Silverman DH, Geist CL, Kenna HA, *et al*, "Differences in regional brain metabolism associated with specific formulations of hormone therapy in postmenopausal women at risk for AD," *Psychoneuroendocrinology*, Aug 30, 2010 (Epub ahead of print).

35. Kublickiene K, "Effects in postmenopausal women of estradiol and medroxyprogesterone alone and combined on resistance artery function and endothelial morphology and movement," *Journal of Clinical Endocrinology and Metabolism*, vol. 93, no. 5 (2008): pp 1874-1883.

36. Cholerton B, Gleason CE, Baker LD, *et al*, "Estrogen and Alzheimer's disease: the story so far," *Drugs & Aging*, vol. 19, no. 6 (2002): pp 405-427.

37. Nilsen J, Brinton RD, "Impact of progestins on estrogen-induced neuroprotection: synergy by progesterone and 19-norprogesterone and antagonism by medroxyprogesterone acetate," *Endocrinology,* vol. 143 (2002): pp 205-212.

38. Nilsen J, Brinton RD, "Effects of estrogen plus progestin on risk of dementia," *Journal of the American Medical Association,* vol. 290, no. 13 (2003): p 1706.

39. Tschanz, JI, Treiber, K., Norton PhD, *et al,* (2005), "A Population Study of Alzheimer's Disease: Findings From the Cache County Study of Memory, Health and Aging," *Case Management Journals,* vol. 6, (2):pp 107-114.

40. Stamm WE, (1993) "A controlled trial of intravaginal estriol in postmenopausal women with recurrent urinary tract infections," *New England Journal of Medicine* :pp 753-756.

41. Brown JS, Vittinghoff E, Kanaya AM, *et al,* (2001) "Urinary tract infections in postmenopausal women: effect of hormone therapy and risk fators," *Obstetrics and Gynecology,* 98(6): pp 1045-1052.

42. Waetjen LE, Brown JS, Vittinghoff E, *et al,* "The effect of ultralow-dose transdermal estradiol on urinary incontinence in postmenopausal women," *Obstetrics and Gynecology,* vol. 106, no. 5 (2005): pp 946-952.

43. Grady D, Brown JS, Vittinghoff E, *et al,* "Postmenopausal hormones and incontinence: the heart and estrogen/progestin replacement study," *Obstetrics and Gynecology,* vol. 97, no. 1 (2001): pp 166-120.

44. Hendrix SL, Cochrane BB, Nygaard IE, *et al,* "Effects of estrogen with and without progestin on urinary incontinence," *Journal of the American Medical Association,* vol. 293, (2005): pp 935-948.

45. Townsend MK, Curhan GC, Resnick NM, *et al,* "Postmenopausal hormone therapy and incident urinary incontinence in middle-aged women," *American Journal of Obstetrics and Gynecology,* vol. 200, no.1 (2009): p 86.

46. Koushik A, *et al,* "Characteristics of menstruation and pregnancy and the risk of lung cancer in women," *International Journal of Cancer,* vol. 125, no. 10 (2009): pp 2428-2433.

47. Guimaraes P, Frisina ST, Mapes F, *et al*, "Progestin negatively affects hearing in aged women," *Proceedings of the National Academy of Sciences of the United States of America*, vol. 103, no. 38 (2006): pp 14246-14249.

Chapter 22 - *The risks of not taking estrogen*

1. Dennison E, Mohamed MA, Cooper C, "Epidemiology of Osteoporosis," *Rheumatic Disease Clinics of North America*, vol. 32, no. 4 (2006): pp 617-780.
2. The Writing Group for the PEPI, "Effects of hormone therapy on bone mineral density: results from the postmenopausal estrogen/progestin interventions (PEPI) trial," *Journal of the American Medical Association*, vol. 276 (1996): p 1389.
3. Prince RL, Smith M, Dick IM, *et al*, "Prevention of postmenopausal osteoporosis: a comparative study of exercise, calcium supplementation, and hormone-replacement therapy," *New England Journal of Medicine*, vol. 325 (1991): p 1189.
4. Field CS, Ory SJ, Wahner HW, *et al*, "Preventive effects of transdermal 17B-estradiol on osteoporotic changes after surgical menopause: a two-year placebo-controlled trial," *American Journal of Obstetrics and Gynecology*, vol. 168 (1993): p 114.
5. Kleppinger A, Kulidorff M, "Ultralow-dose micronized 17 B-estradiol and bone density and bone metabolism in older women," *Journal of the American Medical Association*, vol. 290, no. 8 (2003): pp 1042–1048.
6. Gao Y, Qian W, Dark K, *et al*," Estrogens prevents bone loss through transforming growth Factor Beta signaling in T cells," *Proceedings of the National Academy of Sciences of the United States of America* , vol. 101, no.47 (2004): 16618-16623
7. Banks E, Beral V, Reeves G, *et al*, "Fracture incidence in relation to the pattern of use of hormone therapy in postmenopausal women." *Journal of the American Medical Association*, vol. 291, no. 18 (2004): pp 2212-2220.
8. Lufkin EG, Wahner HW, Judd HL, *et al*, "Treatment of postmenopausal osteoporosis with transdermal estrogen," *Annals of Internal Medicine*, vol. 117, no. 1 (1992): pp 1-9.

9. Villareal DT, Binder EF, Williams DB, *et al,* "Bone mineral density response to estrogen replacement in frail elderly women: a randomized controlled trial," *Journal of the American Medical Association,* vol. 286, no. 7 (2001): pp 815-20.

10. Wimalawansa SJ, "A four-year randomized controlled trial of hormone replacement and bisphosphonate, alone or in combination, in women with postmenopausal osteoporosis," *American Journal of Medicine,* vol. 104, no. 3 (1998): pp 219-226.

11. Odvina CV, Zerwekh JE, Pak CY, *et al,* "Severely suppressed bone turnover: a potential complication of alendronate therapy," *Journal of Clinical Endocrinology and Metabolism,* vol. 90, no. 3 (2005): pp 1294-301.

12. Chen D, Kalu DN, "Modulation of intestinal estrogen receptor by ovariectomy, estrogen and growth hormone," *Pharmacology and Experimental Therapeutics,* vol. 286, no. 1 (1998): pp 328-333.

13. Gao Y, Qian WP, Dark K, *et al,* "Estrogen prevents bone loss through transforming growth factor beta signaling in T cells," *Proceedings of the National Academy of Sciences USA,* vol 101, no. 47 (2004): pp 16618-16623.

14. Ebeling PR, Sandgren MD, DiMagno DP, *et al,* "Evidence of an age-related decrease in intestinal responsiveness to vitamin D: relationship between serum 1,25-dihydroxyvitamin D3 and intestinal vitamin D receptor concentrations in normal women," *Journal of Clinical Endocrinology and Metabolism,* vol. 75, no. 1 (1992): pp 176-182.

15. Gennari C, Agnusdei D, Nardi P, *et al,* "Estrogen preserves a normal intestinal responsiveness to 1,25 dihydroxyvitamin D3 in oophorectomized women," *Journal of Clinical Endocrinology and Metabolism,* vol. 71, no. 5 (1990): pp 1288-1293.

16. Russell JE, Morimoto S, Birge SJ, *et al,* "Effects of age and estrogen on calcium absorption in the rat," *Journal of Bone and Mineral Research,* vol. 1, no. 2 (1986): pp 185-189.

17. Paganini-Hill A, Henderson VW, "Estrogen Deficiency and Risk of Alzheimer's Disease in Women," *American Journal of Epidemiology,* vol. 140, no. 3P (1994): pp 256-261.

18. Plassman BL, Langa KM, Fisher GG, *et al*, "Prevalence of dementia in the United States: The Aging, Demographics, and Memory Study," *Neuroepidemiology*, vol. 29 (2007): pp 125-132.

19. Rosario ER, *et al*, "Progesterone and estrogen regulate Alzheimer-like neuropathology in female 3xTg-AD Mice," *Journal of NeuroScience*, vol. 27, no. 48 (2007): pp 13357-13365.

20. Sherwin B, "Estrogen and cognitive functioning in women," *Endocrine Reviews*, vol. 24, no. 2 (2003): pp 133-151.

21. Tierney M, "Presentation at the International Conference on Alzheimer's disease," August 12, 2008.

22. Smith YR, Love T, *et al*, "Impact of combined estradiol and norethindrone therapy on visuospatial working memory assessed by Functional Magnetic Resonance Imaging," *Journal of Clinical Endocrinology and Metabolism*, vol. 91, no. 11 (2006): pp 4476-4461.

23. Rocca WA, Bower JH, *et al*, "Increased risk of parkinsonism in women who underwent oophorectomy before menopause," *Neurology*, vol. 69 (2007): pp 1074-1083

24. Craig MC, Maki PM, Murphy DGM, " The Women's Health Initiative Memory Study: findings and implications for treatment," *The Lancet (Neurology)*, vol. 4 (2005): pp 1–5.

25. Silverman D and Geist C, (2008) Estrogen May be Neuroprotective After All, *Society of Nuclear Medicine*, 2008 Annual Meeting: Abstract 973, Presented 6-16-08.

26. Cholerton B, Gleason CE, Baker LD, *et al*, "Estrogen and Alzheimer's disease: the story so far," *Drugs & Aging*, vol. 19, no. 6 (2002): pp 405-427.

27. Asthana S, Baker LD, Craft S, *et al*, "High-dose estradiol improves cognition for women with AD," *Neurology*, vol. 57 (2001): pp 605-612.

28. Asthana S, Craft S, Baker LD, *et al*, "Cognitive and neuroendocrine response to transdermal estrogen in postmenopausal women with Alzheimer's disease: results of a placebo-controlled, double-blind, pilot study," *Psychoneuroendocrinology*, vol. 24, no. 6 (1999): pp 657-677.

29. Mulnard RA, Cotman CW, Kawas D, *et al*, "Estrogen replacement therapy for treatment of mild to moderate Alzheimer disease, a randomized controlled trial," *Journal of the American Medical Association*, vol. 283, no. 8 (2000): pp 1007-1015.

30. LeBlanc ES, Janowsky J, *et al*, "Hormone replacement therapy and cognition, systematic review and meta-analysis," *Journal of the American Medical Association*, vol. 285, (2001): pp 1489-1499.

31. Birge SJ, "The use of estrogen in older women," *Clinics in Geriatric Medicine*, vol. 19 (2003): pp 617-627.

32. Tschanz JT, Treiber K, Norton MC, *et al*, "A population study of Alzheimer's disease: findings from the Cache County Study on memory, health, and aging," *Case Management Journals*, vol. 6, no. 2 (2005): pp 107-114.

33. Roussouw JE, Prentice RL, *et al*, "Postmenopausal hormone therapy and risk of cardiovascular disease by age and years since menopause," *Journal of the American Medical Association*, vol. 297 (2007): pp 1465-1477.

34. Mikkola T, Clarkson T, "Estrogen replacement therapy, atherosclerosis and vascular function," *Cardiovascular Research*, vol. 53 (2002): pp 605-619.

35. Lokkegaard E, Andreasen AH, *et al*, "Hormone therapy and risk of myocardial infarction: a national register study," *European Heart Journal*, vol. 29 (2008): pp 2660-2668.

36. Shipra S, Pralhad K, "Effect of menopausal hormone replacement therapy on fibrinogen and antithrombin III levels," *Obstetrics and Gynecology India*, vol. 57, no. 2 (2007) : pp 135-138.

37. Lee AJ, Gordon DO, Lowe W, *et al*, "Plasma fibrinogen in women: relationships with oral contraception, the menopause and hormone replacement," *British Journal of Haematology*, vol. 84, no. 4 (2008): pp 616-621.

38. Decensi A, Omodei U, *et al*, "Effect of transdermal estradiol and oral conjugated estrogen on C-reactive protein in Retinoid-placebo trial in healthy women," *Circulation*, vol. 106 (2002): pp 1224.

39. Godsland IF, "Effects of postmenopausal hormone replacement therapy on lipid, lipoprotein, and apolipoprotein (a) concentrations: analysis of studies published from 1974–2000," *Fertility and Sterility*, vol. 75, no. 5 (2001): pp 898–915.

40. Shifren JL, "A comparison of the short-term effects of oral conjugated equine estrogens versus transdermal estradiol on C-reactive protein, other serum markers of inflammation, and other hepatic proteins in naturally menopausal women," *Journal of Clinical Endocrinology and Metabolism*, vol. 93, no. 5 (2008): pp 1702-1710.

41. Kublickiene K, "Effects in postmenopausal women of estradiol and medroxyprogesterone alone and combined on resistance artery function and endothelial morphology and movement," *Journal of Clinical Endocrinology and Metabolism*, vol. 93, no. 5 (2008): pp 1874-1883.

42. Manson JE, Allison MA, *et al*, "Estrogen Therapy and Coronary-Artery Calcification," *New England Journal of Medicine*, vol. 346, no. 25 (2007): pp 2591-2602.

43. AHA Expert Panel Statement of Prevention V Conference, "Beyond secondary prevention: identifying the high-risk patient for primary prevention: noninvasive tests of atherosclerotic burden: writing group III," *Circulation*, vol. 101 (2000): pp e16-e22.

44. Hurst RT, Daniel WC, Kendall BS, *et al*, "Clinical use of carotid intima-media thickness: review of the literature," *Journal of the American Society of Echocardiography*, vol. 20 (2007): pp 907-914.

45. Hsia J, Langer RD, *et al*, "Conjugated equine estrogens and coronary heart disease," *Archives of Internal Medicine*, vol. 166 (2006): pp 357-365.

46. Manson JE, "The WHI hormone therapy trials: making sense of the evidence," *Menopause Day Keynote Speech Presented at the American Society for Reproductive Medicine 63rd Annual Meeting:* Oct 13-17, 2007 Washington.

47. "NAMS Position Statement," *Menopause*, vol. 15 (2008): pp 584-603.

48. Karim R, Hodis HN, *et al*, "Relationship between serum levels of sex hormones and progression of subclinical atherosclerosis in postmenopausal women," *Journal of Clinical Endocrinology and Metabolism*, vol. 93, no. 1 (2008): pp 131-138.

49. Clarkson TB, "Can women be identified that will derive considerable cardiovascular benefits from postmenopausal estrogen therapy?" *Journal of Clinical Endocrinology and Metabolism*, vol. 93, no. 1 (2008): pp 37-39.

50. Minkin MJ, "Considerations in the choice of oral vs. transdermal hormone therapy: a review," *The Journal of Reproductive Medicine*, vol. 49, no. 4 (2004): pp 311-320.

51. Lobo RA, "Inflammation, coronary artery disease and hormones," *Menopause*, vol. 15, no. 6 (2008): pp 1036-1038.

52. Goodrow GJ, "Predictors of worsening insulin sensitivity in postmenopausal women," *American Journal of Obstetrics and Gynecology*, vol. 194, no. 2 (2006): pp 355-361.

53. Yeboah J, "Effects of estrogen replacement with and without medroxyprogesterone acetate on brachial flow-mediated vasodilator responses in postmenopausal women with coronary artery disease," *American Heart Journal*, vol. 153, no. 3 (2007): pp 439-444.

54. Weiner MG, "Hormone therapy and coronary heart disease in young women," *Menopause*, vol. 15, no. 1 (2008): pp 86-93.

55. Lisabeth LD, Beiser AS, Brown DL, *et al*, "Age at natural menopause and risk of ischemic stroke: the Framingham Heart Study," *Stroke*, vol. 40 (2009): pp 1044-1049.

56. Lewandowski KC, Komorowski J, *et al*, "Effects of hormone replacement therapy type and route of administration on plasma matrix metalloproteinases and their tissue inhibitors in postmenopausal women," *Journal of Clinical Endocrinology and Metabolism*, vol. 91, no. 8 (2006): pp 3123-3130.

57. Prestwood KM, *et al*, "Effects of conjugated equine estrogen in postmenopausal women with hysterectomy," *Journal of the American Medical Association*, vol. 291, no. 14 (2003): pp 1701–1712.

58. Fantl JA, Cardozo L, McClish DK, "Estrogen therapy in the management of urinary incontinence in postmenopausal women: a meta-analysis: first report of the hormones and urogenital therapy committee," *Obstetrics and Gynecology*, vol. 83, no. 1 (1994): pp 12-18.

59. Cardoza L, Bachmann G, *et al*, "Meta-analysis of estrogen therapy in the management of urogenital atrophy in postmenopausal women: Second report of the Hormones and Urogenital Therapy Committee," *Obstetrics & Gynecology*, vol. 92, no. 4, pt. 2 (1998): pp 722-727.

60. Raz R, Stamm WE, "A controlled trial of intravaginal estriol in postmenopausal women with recurrent urinary tract infections," *New England Journal of Medicine*, vol. 329, no. 11 (1993): pp 753-756.

61. Stamm WE, Raz R, "Factors contributing to susceptibility of postmenopausal women to recurrent urinary infections," *Clinical Infectious Diseases*, vol. 28 (1999): pp 723-725.

62. Brown JS, Vittinghoff E, *et al*, "Urinary tract infections in postmenopausal women: effect of hormone therapy and risk factors," *Obstetrics and Gynecology*, vol. 98, no. 6 (2001): pp 1045- 1052.

63. Margolis KL, Bonds DE, Rodabough RJ, *et al*, "Effect of oestrogen plus progestin on the incidence of diabetes in postmenopausal women: results from the Women's Health Initiative hormone trial," *Diabetologia*, vol. 47 (2004): pp 1175–1187.

64. Cagnacci A, Soldani R, Carriero P, *et al*, "Effects of low doses of transdermal 17 beta-estradiol on carbohydrate metabolism in postmenopausal women," *Journal of Clinical Endocrinology and Metabolism*, vol. 74, no. 6 (1992): pp 1396–400.

65. Gaspard UJ, Gottal JM, *et al*, "Postmenopausal changes of lipid and glucose metabolism: a review of their main aspects." *Maturitas*, vol. 21, no. 3 (1995): pp 171–178.

66. Cagnacci A, Tuveri F, Cirillo R, *et al*, "The effect of transdermal 17-beta-estradiol on glucose metabolism of postmenopausal women is evident during the oral but not the intravenous glucose administration," *Maturitas*, vol. 28, no. 2 (1997): pp 163–167.

67. Gabal LL, Goodman-Gruen D, Barrett-Connor E, "The effect of postmenopausal estrogen therapy on the risk of non-insulin-dependent diabetes mellitus," *American Journal of Public Health*, vol. 87, no. 3 (1997): pp 443–445.

68. Hammond CB, Jelovsek FR, Lee KL, *et al*, "Effects of long-term estrogen replacement therapy. I. Metabolic effects," *American Journal of Obstetrics and Gynecology*, vol. 133, no. 5 (1979): 525–536.

69. Rossi R, Origliani G, Modena MG, "Transdermal 17-beta-estradiol and risk of developing type 2 diabetes in a population of healthy, nonobese postmenopausal women," *Diabetes Care*, vol. 27, no. 3 (2004): pp 645–649.

70. Zhang Y, Howard BV, Cowan LD, *et al*, "The effect of estrogen use on levels of glucose and insulin and the risk of type 2 diabetes in American Indian postmenopausal women: the Strong Heart Study," *Diabetes Care*, vol. 25, no. 3 (2002): pp 500–504.

71. Manson JE, Rimm EB, Colditz GA, *et al*, "A prospective study of postmenopausal estrogen therapy and subsequent incidence of non-insulin-dependent diabetes mellitus," *Annals of Epidemiology*, vol. 2, no. 5 (1992): pp 665–673.

72. Andersson B, Mattsson LA, Hahn L, *et al*, "Estrogen replacement therapy decreases hyperandrogenicity and improves glucose homeostasis and plasma lipids in postmenopausal women with noninsulin-dependent diabetes mellitus," *Journal of Clinical Endocrinology and Metabolism*, vol. 82, no. 2 (1997): pp 638-643.

73. Freenan R, "Editorial: Are blood glucose levels affected by menopause?" *Menopause*, vol. 14, no.3 (2007): pp 350-351.

74. Otsuki M, Kasayama S, Morita S, *et al*, "Menopause, but not age, is an independent risk factor for fasting plasma glucose levels in nondiabetic women," *Menopause*, vol. 14, no.3 (2007): pp 404-407.

75. DiCarlo C, Tommaselli GA, *et al*, "Serum leptin levels and body composition in postmenopausal women: effects of hormone therapy," *Menopause*, vol. 11, no. 4 (2004): pp 466-473.

76. Newcomb PA, Storer B, "Postmenopausal hormone use and risk of large bowel cancer," *Journal of National Cancer Institute*, vol. 87 (1995): pp 1067-1071.

77. Kampman E, Potter J, *et al*, "Hormone replacement therapy, reproductive history and colon cancer," *Cancer Causes & Control*, vol. 8 (1997): pp 146–58.

78. Rossouw JE, Anderson GL, *et al*, "Risks and benefits of estrogen plus progestin in healthy postmenopausal women: principal results from the Women's Health Initiative randomized controlled trial," *Journal of the American Medical Association*, vol. 288 (2002): p 321.

79. Grodstein F, Newcomb PA, Stampfer MJ, "Postmenopausal hormone therapy and the risk of colorectal cancer: a review and meta-analysis," *American Journal of Medicine*, vol. 106 (1999): p 574.

80. Ekblad S, Bergendahl A, Enler P, *et al*, "Disturbances in postural balance are common in postmenopausal women with vasomotor symptoms," *Climacteric*, vol. 3, no. 3 (2000): pp 192-198.

81. Hammar ML, Lindgren R, *et al*, "Effects of hormonal replacement therapy on the postural balance among postmenopausal women," *Obstetrics and Gynecology*, vol. 88, no. 6 (1996): pp 955-960.

82. Armstrong AL, Oborne J, *et al*, "Effects of hormone replacement therapy on muscle performance and balance in post-menopausal women," *Clinical Science*, vol. 91, no. 6 (1996): pp 685-690.

83. Ditkoff EC, Crary WG, Lobo RA, "Estrogen improves psychological function in asymptomatic postmenopausal women," *Obstetrics and Gynecology*, vol. 78, no. 6 (1991): pp 991-995.

84. Soares CN, Almeida OP, Joffe H, *et al*, "Efficacy of estradiol for the treatment of depressive disorders in perimenopausal women: a double-blind, randomized, placebo-controlled trial," *Archives of General Psychiatry*, vol. 58, no. 6 (2001): pp 529-534.

85. Rocca WA, Grossardt BR, Geda YE, *et al*, "Long-term risk of depressive and anxiety symptoms after early bilateral oophorectomy," *Menopause*, vol. 15, no. 6 (2008) : pp 1050-1059.

86. Zweifel JE, O'Brien, "A meta-analysis of the effect of hormone replacement therapy upon depressed mood," *Psychoneuroendocrinology*, vol. 22, no. 8 (1997): p 655.

87. Hlatky MA, Boothroyd D, Vittinghoff E, HERS Research Group, "Quality-of-life and depressive symptoms in postmenopausal women after receiving hormone therapy: results from the Heart and Estrogen/Progestin Replacement Study (HERS) trial," *Journal of the American Medical Association*, vol. 287, no.5 (2002): pp 591-597.

88. Carlson CL, Cushman M, Enright PL, *et al*, "Hormone replacement therapy is associated with higher FEV1 in elderly women," *American Journal of Respiratory and Critical Care Medicine*, vol. 163 (2001): pp 423-428.

89. Massaro D, Massaro GD, "Estrogen regulates pulmonary alveolar formation, loss and regeneration in mice," *American Journal of Physiology - Lung Cellular and Molecular Physiology*, vol. 287 (2004): pp L1154-L1159.

90. Massaro GD, Mortola JP, Massaro D, "Estrogen modulates the dimensions of the lung's gas-exchange surface area and alveoli in female rats," *American Journal of Physiology - Lung Cellular and Molecular Physiology*, vol. 270 (1996): pp L110-L114.

91. Massaro D, Massaro GD, "Toward therapeutic pulmonary alveolar regeneration in humans," *Proceedings of the American Thoracic Society*, vol. 3 (2006): pp 709-712.

92. Lim RH, Kobzik L, "Editorial - sexual tension in the airways, the puzzling duality of estrogen in asthma," *American Journal of Respiratory Cell and Molecular Biology*, vol. 38 (2008): pp 499-500.

93. Barr RG, Wentowski CC, *et al*, "Prospective study of postmenopausal hormone use and newly diagnosed asthma and chronic obstructive pulmonary disease," *Archives of Internal Medicine*, vol. 164 (2004): pp 379-386.

94. Feskanich D, Cho E, *et al*, "Menopausal and reproductive factors and risk of age-related macular degeneration," *Archives of Ophthalmology*, vol. 126, no.4 (2008): pp 519-524.

95. Younan C, Mitchell P, Cumming RG, *et al*, "Hormone replacement therapy, reproductive factors, and the incidence of cataract and cataract surgery: the Blue Mountains Eye Study," *American Journal of Epidemiology*, vol. 155, no. 11 (2002): pp 997-1006.

96. Worzala K, Hiller R, Sperduto RD, *et al*, "Postmenopausal estrogen use, type of menopause, and lens opacities: the Framingham studies," *Archives of Internal Medicine*, vol. 161 (2001): p 1448.

97. Freeman EE, Munoz B, Schein OD, *et al*, "Hormone replacement therapy and lens opacities: the Salisbury Eye Evaluation project," *Archives of Ophthalmology*, vol. 119 (2001): p 1687.

98. Speroff L and Fritz MA, Editors: *Clinical Gynecologic Endocrinology and Infertility*, 7th Edition (2004): p 753.

99. Kilicdag EB, Yavuz H, Bagis T, "Effects of estrogen therapy on hearing in postmenopausal women," *American Journal of Obstetrics and Gynecology*, vol. 190, no. 1 (2004): pp 77-82.

100. Morimoto N, Tanaka T, Horikawa R, *et al*, "Hearing loss in Turner Syndrome," *Journal of Pediatrics*, vol. 149 (2006): pp 697-701.

101. Tezal M, *et al*, "Periodontal disease and the incidence of tooth loss in postmenopausal women," *Journal of Periodontology*, vol. 76, no. 7 (2005): pp 1123-1128.

102. Friedlander AH, "Physiology, medical management and oral implications of menopause," *The Journal of the American Dental Association*, vol. 133, no. 1 (2002): pp 73-81.

103. Paganini-Hill A, "The benefits of estrogen replacement on oral health: the leisure world cohort," *Archives of Internal Medicine*, vol. 155 (1995): p 2325.

104. Krall EA, Dawson-Hughes B, Hannan MT, *et al*, "Postmenopausal estrogen replacement and tooth retention," *American Journal of Medicine*, vol. 102 (1997): p 536.

105. Civitelli R, Pilgram TK, Dotson M, *et al*, "Alveolar and postcranial bone density in postmenopausal women receiving hormone/estrogen replacement therapy," *Archives of Internal Medicine*, vol. 162 (2002): pp 1409-1410.

106. Wolff EF, *et al*, "Long-term effects of hormone therapy on skin rigidity and wrinkles," *Fertility and Sterility*, vol. 84 (2005): pp 285-288.

107. Kaatz M, Elsner P, Koehler MJ, "Changes in skin topography during hormone therapy," *Menopause*, vol. 15, no. 6 (2008): p 1193.

108. Baran R and Maibach HI, Editors: *Textbook of Cosmetic Dermatology* 2nd edition, Taylor & Francis, (1998) pp 489-490.

109. Raine-Fenning NJ, Brincat MP, Muscat-Baron Y, "Skin aging and menopause: implications for treatment," *American Journal of Clinical Dermatology*, vol. 4, no. 6 (2003): pp 371-378.

110. Holland EF, Studd JW, Mansell JP, *et al*, "Changes in collagen composition and cross-links in bone and skin of osteoporotic postmenopausal women treated with percutaneous estradiol implants," *Obstetrics and Gynecology*, vol. 83 (1994): p 180.

111. Maheux R, Naud F, Rioux M, *et al*, "A randomized, double-blind, placebo-controlled study on the effect of conjugated estrogens on skin thickness," *American Journal of Obstetrics and Gynecology*, vol. 170 (1994): p 642.

112. Ashcroft GS, Dodsworth J, van Boxtel E, *et al*, "Estrogen accelerates cutaneous wound healing associated with an increase in TGF-B1," *Natural Medicine*, vol. 3 (1997): p 1209.

113. Verdier-Sévrain S, Bonté F, Gilchres B, "Biology of estrogens in skin: implications for skin aging," *Experimental Dermatology*, vol. 15, no. 2 (2005): pp 83-94.

114. Nevitt MC, Cummings SR, Lane NE, *et al*, "Association of estrogen replacement therapy with the risk of osteoarthritis of the hip in elderly white women," *Archives of Internal Medicine*, vol. 156 (1996): p 2073.

115. Zhang Y, McAlindon TE, Hannan MT, *et al*, "Estrogen replacement therapy and worsening of radiographic knee osteoarthritis," *Arthritis & Rheumatism*, vol. 41 (1998): p 1867.

116. Hak AE, Curhan G, Grodstein FD, *et al*, "Menopause, postmenopausal hormone use and risk of incident gout," *Annals of Rheumatic Diseases,* Vol 69, no. 7 ((2010): pp 1305-1309.

117. Eliassen AH, Missmer SA, *et al*, "Circulating levels of 2-hydroxy and 16-hydroxy estrone levels and risk of breast cancer," *Cancer Epidemiology, Biomarkers & Prevention,* vol. 17 (2008): pp 2029-2035.

118. Im A, Vogel VG, Ahrendt ST, *et al*, "Urinary estrogen metabolites in patients at high risk for breast cancer," *Journal of Clinical Oncology,* vol. 26 (2008): p 1520.

119. Vogel VG, *"Management of Patients at High Risk for Breast Cancer,"* Blackwell Science, Inc, Malden, MA (2001).

120. Davison S and Davis SR, "New markers for cardiovascular disease risk in women: Endogenous estrogen status and exogenous postmenopausal hormone therapy," *Journal of Clinical Endocrinology & Metabolism,* vol. 88, no. 6 (2003): pp 2470-2478.

121. Blum CA, Muller B, Huber P, *et al*, "Low-grade inflammation and estimates of insulin resistance during the menstrual cycle in lean and overweight women," *Journal of Clinical Endocrinology & Metabolism,* vol. 90 (2006): pp 3230-3235.

Section 4 - If you have decided to take HRT, which one to choose?

1. Howell N, Dykens J, "Alzheimer's disease, estrogens and clinical trials: a case study in drug development for complex disorders," *Drug Development Research,* vol. 66, no. 2 (2006): pp 53-77.

2. Magnusson C, Baron JA, Correia N, *et al*, "Breast-cancer risk following long-term oestrogen - and oestrogen-progestin-replacement therapy," *International Journal of Cancer,* vol. 81, no. 3 (1999): pp 339-344.

3. Naunton M, Asmar FY, *et al*, "Estradiol gel: review of the pharmacology, pharmacokinetics, efficacy and safety in menopausal women," *Menopause,* vol. 13 (2006): pp 517-527.

4. Slater CC, Hodis HN, Mack WJ, *et al*, "Markedly elevated levels of estrone sulfate after long-term oral, but not transdermal, administration of estradiol in postmenopausal women," *Menopause,* vol. 8, no. 3 (2001): pp 200-203.

5. Johnson JV, Lowell J, Badger GJ, *et al*, "Effects of oral and transdermal hormonal contraption on vascular risk markers: a randomized controlled trial," *Obstetrics and Gynecology*, vol. 111, no. 2 (2008): pp 278-284.

6. Jensen J, Burke A, Banhart K, *et al*, "Effects of switching from oral to transdermal or transvaginal contraception on markers of thrombosis," *Contraception*, vol. 78, no. 6 (2009) : pp 451-458.

7. Turgeon JL, Carr MC, *et al*, "Complex actions of sex steroids in adipose tissue, the cardiovascular system and brain: insights from basic science and clinical studies," *Endocrine Reviews*, vol. 27, no. 6 (2006): pp 575-605.

8. de Ziegler D, Ferriani R, *et al*, "Vaginal progesterone in menopause: Crinone 4% in cyclical and constant combined regimens," *Human Reproduction*, vol. 15, no. 1 (2000) : pp 149-158.

9. Lobo RA, "Progestogens: the misunderstood component of menopausal hormone therapy," *Progestogen Primer, Menopause Management*, vol. 18 (Suppl1) (2008): pp 3-5.

10. Gillet JY, Andre G, *et al*, "Induction of amenorrhea during hormone replacement therapy: optimal micronized progesterone dose. A multicenter study," *Maturitas*, vol. 19, no. 2 (1994): pp 103-115.

11. Women's Health Initiative Branch, "Postmenopausal hormone therapy and risk of cardiovascular disease by age and years since menopause," *Journal of the American Medical Association*, vol. 297, no. 13 (2007): pp 1465-1467.

12. Shapiro S, "Recent epidemiological evidence relevant to the clinical management of the menopause," *Climacteric*, (suppl 2) (2007): pp 2-15.

13. Colditz GA, Manson JE, Hankinson SE, "The Nurses Health Study: 20 year contribution to the understanding of health among women," *Journal of Women's Health*, vol. 6, no. 1 (1997): pp 49-62.

14. Chlebowski R, Kuller L, Prentice R, *et al*, "Breast cancer after use of estrogen plus progestin in postmenopausal women," *New England Journal of Medicine*, vol. 360 (2009): pp 573-587.

15. Somboonporn W and Davis SR, "Postmenopausal testosterone therapy and breast cancer risk," *Maturitas*, vol. 49 (2004): pp 267-275.

16. Dimitrakakis D, Zhou J, Wang J, *et al*, "A physiologic role for testosterone in limiting estrogenic stimulation of the breast," *Menopause*, vol. 10, no. 4 (2003): pp 292-298.

17. Somboonporn W, Davis SR, "Testosterone effects on the breast: implications for testosterone therapy for women," *Endocrine Reviews*, vol. 25, no. 3 (2004): pp 374-388.

18. Key T, Appleby P, Barnes I, Reeves G, "Endogenous sex hormones and breast cancer in postmenopausal women: reanalysis of nine prospective studies," *Journal of National Cancer Institute*, vol. 94, no. 8 (2002): pp 606-616.

19. Kaaks R, Berrino F, Key T, *et al*, "Serum sex steroids in premenopausal women and breast cancer risk within the European Prospective Investigation into Cancer and Nutrition (EPIC)," *Journal of National Cancer Institute*, vol. 97, no. 10 (2005): pp 755-765.

20. Micheli AM, Meneghini E, Secreto G, *et al*, "Plasma testosterone and prognosis of postmenopausal breast cancer patients," *Journal of Clinical Oncology*, vol. 24, no. 19 (2007): pp 2685-2690.

21. Tamimi RM, Byrne C, *et al*, "Endogenous hormone levels, mammographic density and subsequent risk of breast cancer in postmenopausal women," *Journal of National Cancer Institute*, vol. 99 (2007): pp 1178-1187.

22. Eliassen AH, Missmer SA, *et al*, "Endogenous steroid hormone concentrations and risk of breast cancer: does the association vary by a woman's predicted breast cancer risk?," *Journal of Clinical Oncology*, vol. 24, no. 12 (2006): pp 1823-1830.

23. Vogel VG, Taioli, E, "Have we found the ultimate risk factor for breast cancer?," *Journal of Clinical Oncology*, vol. 24, no. 12 (2006): pp 1791-1794.

24. Morrow M, Jordan VC, editors, *Managing Breast Cancer Risk*, BC Decker Inc, Lewisville NY, 2003, p 49.

25. Fournier A, Berrino F, *et al*, "Breast cancer risk in relation to different types of hormone replacement therapy in the E3N-EPIC cohort," *International Journal of Cancer*, vol. 114 (2005): pp 448-454.

26. Fournier A, Berrino F, Clavel-Chapelon F, "Unequal risks for breast cancer associated with different hormone replacement therapies: results from the E3N cohort study," *Breast Cancer Research and Treatment*, vol. 107, no. 1 (2008): pp 103-111.

27. Karim R, "Relationship between serum levels of sex hormones and progression of subclinical atherosclerosis in postmenopausal women," *Journal of Clinical Endocrinology and Metabolism*, vol. 93, no. 1 (2008): pp 131-138.

28. Miller VM, Duckles SP, "Vascular actions of estrogens: functional implications," *Pharmacological Reviews*, vol. 60 (2008): pp 210-224.

29. Labrie F, Luu-the V, Labrie C, *et al*, "Endocrine and intracrine sources of androgens in women: inhibition of breast cancer and other roles of androgens and their precursor dehydroepiandrosterone," *Endocrine Reviews*, vol. 24, no. 2 (2003): pp 152-182.

30. Archer DF, "Tailoring progestogen therapy to the individual patient," *Menopause Management*, vol. 18 (Suppl 1) (2009): pp 5-7.

31. Jessel RH, Nachtigall MJ, Nachtigall LE, "Obstetrics and Gynecology, NYU School of Medicine, New York, NY, two cases of endometrial adenocarcinoma in postmenopausal women on bioidentical hormone replacement therapy," Clinical Poster Presentation at the 20th Annual Meeting of the North American Menopause Society Annual Meeting, October 2009.

32. de Ziegler D, Ferriani R, *et al*, "Vaginal progesterone in menopause: Crinone 4% in cyclic and constant combined regimens," *Human Reproduction*, vol. 15, no. 1 (2000): pp 149-158.

33. Patel SM, Ratcliffe SJ, Reilly MP, *et al*, "Higher serum testosterone concentration in older women is associated with insulin resistance, metabolic syndrome, and cardiovascular disease," *Journal of Clinical Endocrinology and Metabolism*, vol. 94, no. 12 (2009): pp 4776-4784.

34. Janssen I, Powell LH, Crawford S, *et al*, "Menopause and the metabolic syndrome the Study of Women's Health Across the Nation (SWAN)," *Archives of Internal Medicine,* vol. 168, no. 14 (2008): pp 1568-1575.

35. Kraemer GR, Kraemer RR, Ogden BW, *et al*, "Variability of serum estrogens among postmenopausal women treated with the same transdermal estrogen therapy and the effect on androgens and sex hormone binding globulin," *Fertility and Sterility,* vol. 79, no. 3 (2003): pp 534-542.

36. Jarvinen A, Nykanen S, Paasiniemi L, "Absorption and bioavailability of oestradiol from a gel, a patch and a tablet," *Maturitas,* vol. 32, no. 2 (1999): pp 103-113.

37. Reginstera JY, Alberta A, Deroisya R, *et al*, "Plasma estradiol concentrations and pharmacokinetics following transdermal application of Menorest 50 or System (Evorel) 50," *Maturitas,* vol. 27, no. 2 (1997): pp 179-286.

38. Jarvinen A, Backstrom AC, Elfstrom C, *et al*, "Comparative absorption and variability in absorption of estradiol from a transdermal gel and a novel matrix-type transdermal patch," *Maturitas,* vol. 38, no. 2 (2001): pp 189-196.

39. Lewis JG, McGill H, Patton VM, *et al*, "Caution on the use of saliva measurements to monitor absorption of progesterone from transdermal creams in postmenopausal women," *Maturitas,* vol. 41, no. 1 (2002): pp 1-6.

Section 5 - Afterward - Seeing the big picture and the cycle of life

1. Ray NF, Chan JK, Thamer M, *et al*, "Medical expenditures for the treatment of osteoporotic fractures in the United States in 1995: report from the National Osteoporosis Foundation," *Journal of Bone and Mineral Research,* vol. 12 (1997): pp 24-35.

2. National Osteoporosis Foundation, "Osteoporosis fast facts," www.nof.org/osteoporosis/diseasefacts.htm Accessed March 21, 2009.

3. Alzheimer's Association, "2008 Alzheimer's disease facts and figures," www.alz.org/alzheimers_disease_facts_figures.asp Accessed March 21, 2009.

4.   Lloyd-Jones D, Adams R, Carnethon M, *et al*, "Heart disease and stroke statistics 2009 update: a report from the American Heart Association Statistics Committee and Stroke Statistics Subcommittee," *Circulation*, vol. 119 (2008): pp e21-e181.

5.   Fries JF, Koop CE, *et al*, "Reducing health care costs by reducing the need and demand for medical services," *New England Journal of Medicine*, vol. 329, no. 5 (1993): pp 321-325.

6.   Vita AJ, Terr RB, Hubert HB, *et al*, "Aging, health risks and cumulative disability," *New England Journal of Medicine*, vol. 338, no. 15 (1998): pp 1035-1041.

7.   Editorial, "Aging better," *New England Journal of Medicine*, vol. 338, no. 15 (1998): pp 1064-1066.

Index